Best New Natural Weight Loss Program: Large Print

"Discover how easy it is to lose weight naturally"

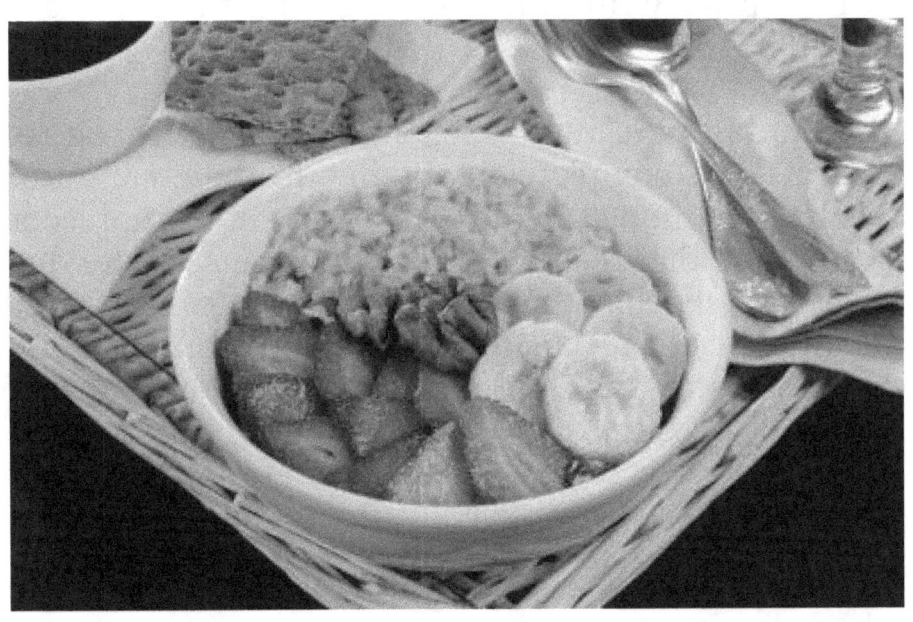

Rudy S. Silva, Natural Nutritionist

ISBN-13: 978-1508413646
ISBN-10: 1508413649

Disclaimer and Terms of Use:

The Author and Publisher have strived to be as accurate and complete as possible in the creation of this book, although he does not warrant or represent at any time that the contents within are accurate due to the rapidly changing nature of the Internet. While all attempts have been made to verify information provided in this publication, the Author and Publisher assume no responsibility for errors, omissions, or contrary interpretation of the subject matter herein. Any perceived slights of specific persons, peoples, or organizations are unintentional.

All readers are advised to seek their own medical help.

The information here is for educational purposes and in no way is it medical advice or treatment. Ask your doctor before using any of the natural remedies listed here.

Table of Contents

1: Introduction To Weight Loss

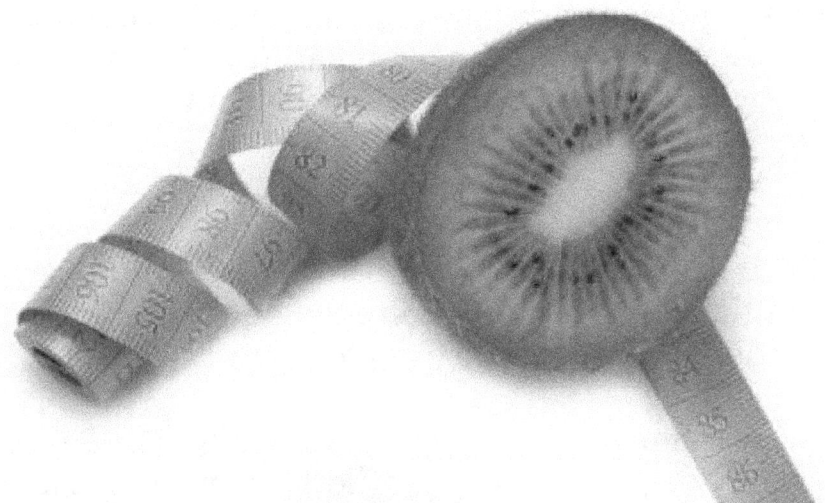

Who I Am and Why I Can Help You

I'm Rudy Silva, Natural Nutritionist, educated at the Bauman School of Holistic Nutrition. I have over 45 kindle books and physical books on Nutrition and Natural Remedies.

I have been in the Nutrition field since 1997 and worked with individual with a variety of ailments and body conditions. During this time, I have notice the way people eat that leads them into illness and obesity.

As I helped people get over the various body conditions, I have gathered and developed the best ideas and methods for losing weight. I have seen various weight-loss programs come and go, but there is still only one basic principle that underlines losing weight – eating fewer calories than your body needs and eating highly nutritious food.

The weight-loss program I have here for you is using the best nutritional ideas and eating natural food. In some cases certain metabolic boosters are advised to accelerate your weight loss.

If you are interested in discovering how you can adjust your eating habits to lose weight and at the same time elevate your health, using natural food and nutrition, this is the program for you.

If you want to lose weight quickly, for whatever reason, then you need another program. Most lose weight fast programs work for a short time, but not for a life time. In this program, you will learn how and why to eat right. When you start eating the way your body wants you to eat, you not only lose weight but you become healthier.

I'm not telling you that it is easy to change your eating habits. Changing habits of any kind is difficult to do and can be done is a reasonable time. As you learn how and when to eat nutritious foods you like, you will develop your own natural way of eating.

So join me and others in finally using a weight-loss program that makes sense, using natural food and nutrition.

2: Why You Should Want To Lose Weight

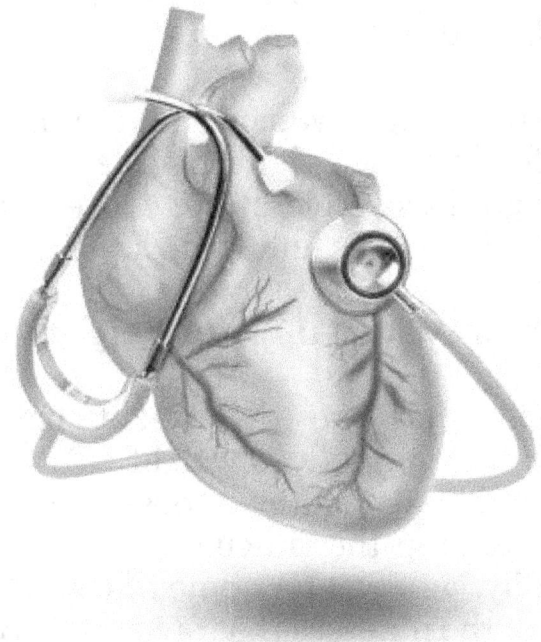

In this book, you will get the best information about how you can lose weight naturally. No pill here that you need to take for months on end. You will get a ton of weight loss information that works. From this, you can create a natural way of eating, so that you can maintain and control your weight, when you wish.

This information here can be overwhelming at first, but at the end of this book, I give you a complete step by step sample program. You can use this sample program to develop your own weight-loss program, using the natural foods listed here or the ones you like to eat.

Losing weight is all about the amount of calories you eat, and that you burn. You can't lose weight simply by taking some pill and eating what you want. But, you can use some natural weight-loss pills, which are called weight loss accelerator; this program will list them in a later chapter.

So, reduce the calories you eat, eat the right foods, eat the right foods at the right time, exercise, and use natural weight loss accelerators to lose weight. In this book, you will discover how to do all of this naturally.

Why Do You Want To Lose Weight?

Most people that are overweight have different reasons for wanting to lose weight. For some, it's to look good and to attract the opposite sex. For others, it could be to stop the ridicule and gross comments received daily. And yet for some others, it could be to stop some of the illnesses that favor obesity.

But, whatever reason you have for wanting to trim down, what you will walk away with when you get into this eating habit program will be less weight. And, you will have some of the best health you have ever had.

Losing weight, you have found, is not easy, but it does not have to be complicated, so you need a diet or an eating habit that you can keep using, after your diet period is over. You don't need a weight-loss program that you do and after you finish it, you later gain the weight back.

When you strive to gain the best health, you have ever had, you will lose weight. Excess weight and health do not go together. When you have too much weight on your body, you are over working all the organs inside your body and reducing their life time. What this does is encourage disease that doesn't necessarily show up right away, but shows up slowly, as you age.

Most people over 40 and even sooner start to experience disease that requires a doctor's intervention, hospitalization, or drug therapy. If you are overweight, you can expect to be ill, as time passes. Being overweight brings untold damage to your body and your life time is reduced substantially.

Is It Your Fault That You Are Overweight?

Yes, it may be that this is the case. But, being overweight has many causes, and sometimes it may not be your fault you are overweight. If you have a genetic marker that predisposes you to excess weight, then the information here will help you to control your own life.

If you come from an overweight family that allowed you to over eat junk and fatty foods as you grew up, then you need to work, as an adult, to reverse those eating habits.

If you have thyroid issues, then your metabolism may be altered, causing you to gain weight. Before you start this program, you might want to get your thyroidal function checked.

Now, there are many cases where it is your fault that you are overweight. You decide what food that you want and need to eat. If you are eating more calories than you need to keep your body working as it should, those calories will be stored as excess fat.

3: How To Lose Weight Program

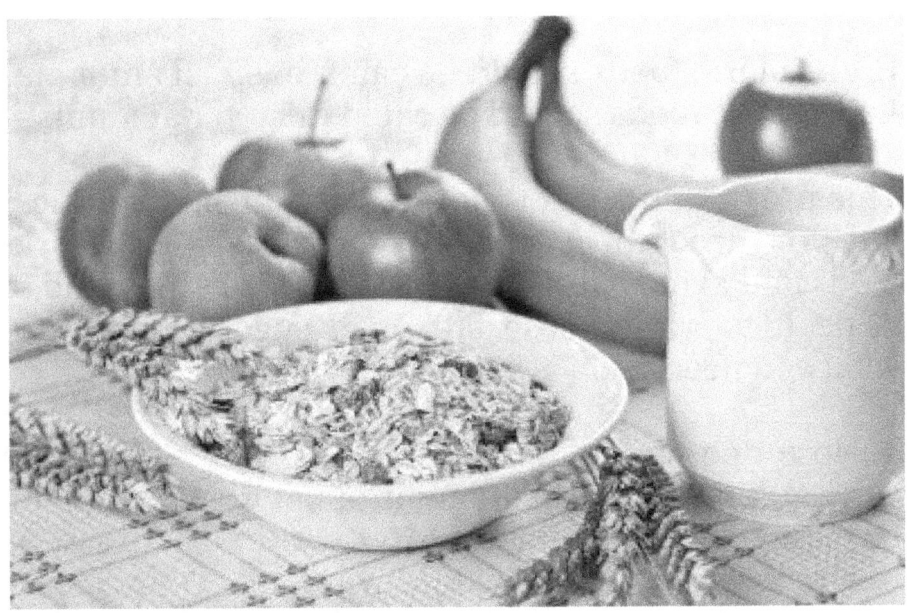

How To Lose Weight

Most people that are overweight eat the wrong kind of food. The food they eat does not provide them with the right nutrition and energy. They over eat fattening food, over cooked food, processed food, fast food, and food in packages and cans.

All of these types of food are high in calories, but lack the right nutrients that the body needs. When you eat food, you should be aware of which foods are high in calories, so that you don't eat more calories than your body needs.

In this program, you need to reduce your calorie intake by 500 to 1000 calories, but you don't want to go below 1300 calories. You only need to do this for a few weeks.

High-calorie foods should be eaten in small amounts. Low calorie foods should be eaten in larger amounts.

This program does not require you to count calories, but you need to be of aware of those high-calorie foods and avoid eating them. At first, you may find it difficult to avoid those fatty and sugary foods, but what you need to do is start cutting back on them.

To lose one pound, you need to reduce the calories you eat by 3400. The amount of calories you might be eating, as a woman, is 1800 to 2000 calories. So, reducing your calories by 500 will move your calorie intake to 1300 to 1500. This is what you should plan for.

For men, you might be eating 2000 to 2500 calories per day, so you need to back off to 1500 to 2000 per day.

To make sure you remain healthy, you should not go below consuming 1200 calories per day. This program will provide this amount of calories or more so that you can start losing weight naturally. The more you apply this program, the more weight you will in a healthy manner.

In This Program

You will be eating protein from fish, chicken, and red meat. You need to eat the right amount of meat to lose weight. But, you also have to reduce the amount of high calorie carbohydrates.

Then, you have to eat special basic soups, vegetables, fruits, nuts, grains and brown rice listed here.

Protein

To lose weight, you need to eat good protein. You may not need to eat more than 3 ounces of meat or 60 gm. per day. Your protein needs will depend upon the type of work you do. If you are an office worker, are short and have a small body frame, you may only need 2 or 3 oz. of meat per day. But, if you are a husky man with a large bone structure and have a physical job, then you may need 12 oz. of meat per day or more.

Quality protein is going to give you the vitality and energy your body needs. The amino acids in the protein will provide the amines needed to create the enzymes you need to control your cell metabolism properly. Good cell metabolism is needed, so that you can control your weight.

Any weight-loss program that limits meat from your diet will fail to help you lose weight and to keep it off.

The Fiber Factor

By adding the right amount and quality fiber to this eating habit program, you bring in a new factor for losing weight. The combination of protein and quality fiber at each meal will improve your success in losing weight with this eating habit program.

Fiber is one of the main factors in losing weight, since it has tremendous health benefits and is a major factor in whether you can lose weight and can keep it off.

Fiber does not contain calories. It is an indigestible nutrient that exists in carbohydrates that gives you bulk, a feeling of fullness, and helps you lose weight.

You need to eat a high amount of fiber, between 30 to 45 gram and an average of 37 grams per day.

Disease
If you are overweight, you, mostly likely, will be fighting some illness or disease. This program helps to improve your health and weight.

If you have constipation, this weight-loss program will eliminate it. If you have diabetes, this program will help you stabilize your sugar levels. If you have acid reflux or arthritis, this program will help you decrease your symptoms or even eliminate these conditions. This goes to show how critical it is to be the correct weight and eat those foods that give you nutrition and vitality.

Reducing Toxins

This program is designed so that you can flush out toxins that are throughout your body and deep into your cells. If you have high or low blood pressure, your pressure will start to stabilize. If you suffer from diabetes and many other illnesses, this program will help you reduce the effects of these illnesses.

So, how can such an eating habits program produce all of these results? When you move to follow a more natural way of eating and living, then the illnesses that you have created will lessen. With this eating habits program, you can also expect to move to your natural weight and health.

4: How To Lose Weight In This Program

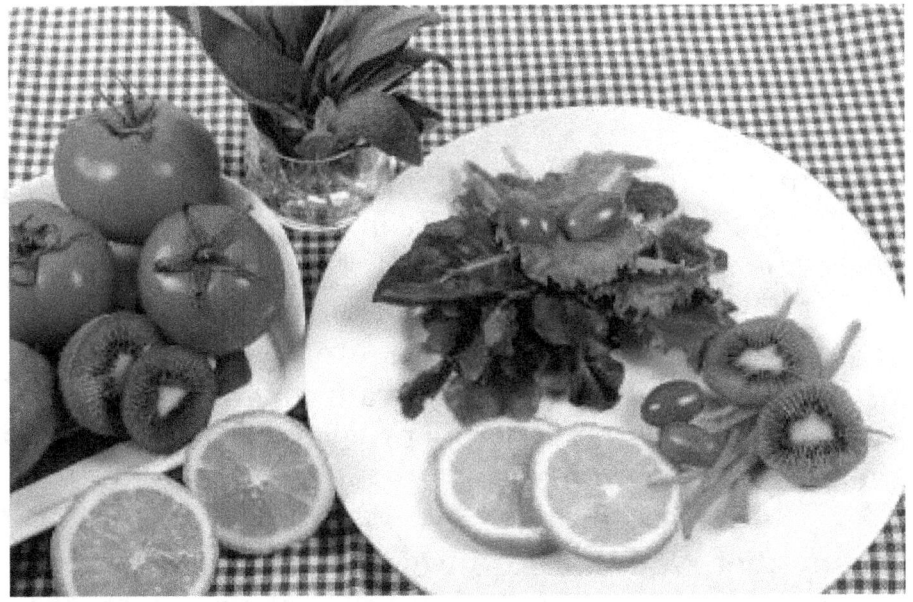

What To Expect From This Program

There are certain weight loss principles that you need to know about. It is these principles that you will be exposed to, and that you can apply to lose and control your weight. This program shows you a healthy way to eat that you can use or expand on, so that it becomes your way of eating all the time.

You will be applying each of these principles little by little. The rate that you apply them will depend on you and where you are in your own health program. If you are already eating somewhat healthy, then you will just need to make some other adjustments.

If you need plenty of help on how to eat to have a healthy body, then you will have a lot of work to do. However, you do not have to do it in one or two weeks or even in one month.

Take it slow, because it took you some time to gain the weight you have. So, start slowly and get rid of it.

The amount of weight that you lose each week will be different for each person. Even so, the best way to work this program is to concentrate on changing your eating habits and using the program as outlined. The weight will start to come off, and you don't have worry about whether the program is working or not. Just start eating the way this program shows you, and the weight will come off.

In any diet, you can lose weight. But, there always seems to be a problem after the diet where 90% of dieters gain their weight back in a year. It won't happen with this way of eating, and when you see some weight creeping in you can make minor changes in your diet.

There is a lot of information here and this can be confusing, so just start adding changes slowly from the different steps and when you feel comfortable add more changes.

Here is the program that you can use to help you get started.

A Natural Eating Habit Lifestyle

- Colon And Body Cleanse

- Using Body Cycles To Lose Weight

- Acid Alkaline Body Weight Loss

- Using Fiber To Lose Weight

- Using Metabolic Enhancers

- Supplements You Should Use

- Exercise For Weight Loss

- Making Smoothies For Weight Loss

Step 1: Colon and body cleanse

In chapter 2, we covered how to do a colon and body cleanse. This is an important cleanse to do since it starts your process of losing weight, by helping you get rid of some of your body toxins, acids, water, fat. This cleanse should be done at least two times a year. Here's what this cleanse does:

- Cleans out your colon of any toxins
- Helps to get your bowel movements back to normal
- Removes some toxins from your cells and lymph liquid
- Removes excess water from your body
- Moves your body away from an acid body making it more alkaline

- Uses some of your fat to provide you with energy during your cleanse.

Step 2 – Using Your Body Cycles

There are three different body cycles your body goes through, and they cover morning, lunch, and dinner.

Morning

Once you finish your cleanse, you are ready to start your new eating pattern. Using the Body Cycles will help you detoxify your body daily, lose weight, keep your weight off, and improve your health.

This cycle is from the time you get up to noon time. During this time, you only want to eat fruits and vegetables and drink juices and teas. This cycle helps you get rid of toxins that your body has accumulated during the night. It does this by urine and bowel movements. You can help your body by providing liquid and nutrients to help detoxify it.

Lunch

Noon is the time to eat heavy food. It is this food that is going to give you the nutrients to provide your body with energy and to help it regenerate itself.

For lunch, you only want to eat enough food for your daily needs. When you eat more than what your body needs to keep it going, it will turn the excess into fat.

After Lunch Snack

Use the ideas given for Morning Snacks for your afternoon snacks.

Notice that you can eat many foods that you cannot in other diets. When you eat foods that you like, do it in small quantities. It's the excess quantity of good and bad foods that you eat that make you fat.

Learn to eat less of the foods you like and eat more frequently. Always eat something during morning and afternoon snack time.

Dinner time

This is the time to eat carbohydrates or more protein. It is best to eat carbohydrates with vegetables and no protein. You may find this hard to do but here is what to eat at dinner time. Eating carbohydrates and protein at the same time make it hard for your stomach to digest this food. The result is poor digestion causing you to crave food before your next meal.

After Dinner Snacks

Try not to eat anything 2 to 3 hours before bedtime. If you need a snack, here is a starter list.

Acid Alkaline Body Weight Loss

Here is another secret in losing weight. You want to

eat those foods that make your body more alkaline. Most people eat more acid food than alkaline food, and this makes their body acidic. An accumulation of acids in your body leads to more weight and disease. In the following chapter, you will learn how to change your body into an alkaline condition, so that your body weight will begin to change.

Using Fiber to Lose Weight

Using fiber information is critical to this weight-loss program. Without using fiber the right way, you will not be able to lose weight or become healthier.

Here is what you need to know about fiber and losing weight.

In this program, you need to build up your fiber intake to 30 to 45 grams. It is at this level that many clinical studies have discovered many of the ideas that will be discussed here. So, 37 grams of fiber are what you need to shoot for.

When you eat fiber foods, your appetite for food will be reduced. This will allow you to reduce that amount of food you eat. So, fiber is an appetite suppressant. You are going to learn what foods contain the most fiber and when to eat these foods.

Using Metabolic Enhancers

Your metabolism determines how fast you burn the food you eat. You want to have a fast metabolism, so that the excess food you eat does not turn into fat. If you have a slow metabolism, your cells will take longer to burn the nutrients you eat, and you will lose weight slower.

There are certain foods and nutrients that you can add to your diet to make your metabolism more active, and thereby helping you to lose weight.

Supplements You Should Use

In any weight loss or health program, there always mineral and vitamins you need to take to make sure you stay or become healthy. By adding these supplements to your diet you will enhance the digestion and absorption of the foods that you eat.

Exercise for Weight Loss

There is no way you can lose weight and stay healthy without exercise. This is one of the other keys to maintaining your weight and health. The exercise you do is unlike what you needed to do in the past. By just exercising for 20 minutes, in a different way, you can achieve your goal of exercise for weight loss and cardiovascular health.

Making Smoothies for Weight Loss

Making smoothies is a fun way to look forward to what you eat. Smoothies can be packed with energy, metabolic enhancers, and acid neutralizers. Drinking them every day is a great way to start the day.

Discover in the next chapters how to make smoothies that encompass all the weight loss ideas presented here.

In the following chapters, you get the information on how and why to do each of the above steps. At the end of this book, a more detail step by step program is provided.

5: Colon Body Cleanse That Accelerate Weight Loss

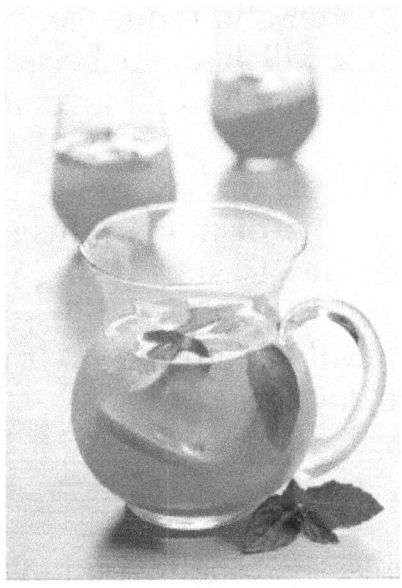

Three to Five Day Cleansing

You will start this weight-loss program right away by doing this colon-body cleanse. While you are doing this 3 day cleanse, you can continue reading the rest of this book. This will quickly allow you to get started on this program.

Starting this cleanse is an important step in your weight program, because you want to remove toxins and mucus from your intestinal tract – stomach, small intestine, and colon. You want to pull out acids that hide in your cells, lymph liquid, muscles or fat cells.

This cleanse will also clean out your blood and neutralize many of the acids in your body that are causing you harm. The cleanse will, in addition, pull out excess body water and reduce any edema that you might have. This will happen because this cleanse promotes urination and bowel movements.

The combination of toxins, acid, and water can weight from 5 to 7 lbs. or more. This colon and blood cleanse is a great way to start losing weight. You can do this cleanse for three days, but if you do it for four to five days, you will benefit more. It is not that hard to do it for three days.

Constipation

Part of this cleanse is to help you have regular bowel movements. If you do not have one to two bowel movements per day, your body will be toxic. Some toxins are often converted to fat. Other toxins are stored in your fat cells. Having regular bowel movements, helps to keep your body clean of toxins, and helps you to keep your weight down.

To help you clear out your colon, there are two ways to do this in this cleanse. You can take Oxypowder, during your three day cleanse, or you can drink prune juice instead.

In this cleanse, you will only be drinking vegetable

juices, fruit juices and eating some fruits for three days. Doing a juice cleanse can give you some side effects, where you feel nauseated or slightly sick.

Not everyone will get these effects. If you feel sick, this is a sign that you are stirring up toxins in your stomach and elsewhere in your body. As you get rid of these toxins, you will begin to feel better.

In her extensive book, Cooking For Healthy Healing, 1991, Linda Rector-page, N.D., Ph.D., talks about what a fast does, "Fasting works by self-digestion. During a cleanse, the body in its infinite wisdom, will decompose and burn only the substances and tissue that are damaged, diseased, or unneeded, such as abscesses, tumors, excess fat deposits, and congestive wastes. Even a relatively short fast can accelerate elimination from the liver, kidneys, lungs and skin, often causing dramatic changes as masses of accumulated waste is expelled. Live foods and juices can literally pick up dead matter from the body and carry it away."

So, here's what you need to do to get started.

The Day Before The Cleanse

Buy the following juices for this cleanse a few days before, or the day before your cleanse.

- Organic apple juice – one gallon

- Organic apples – 3 for one day, 10 apples for 3 days

- Organic prune juice – 1/2 gallon

- Organic Cherry juice – 1/2 gallon

- Carrots for your juicer or carrot juice – one quart

The day before the fast, eat a large salad and two apples at dinner time. This will give you plenty of fiber to scrub the walls of your colon as you move fecal matter out of your colon the following day.

Cleansing The Colon

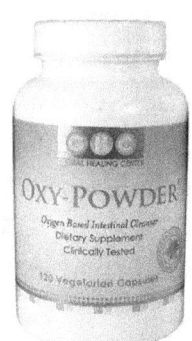

If you choose to use Oxy-Powder, then here is where you can buy it on the Internet:

Get Oxy-Powder

The night before you start your weight loss program, take four Oxy-Powder capsules. If you need to lose a lot of weight, then take five capsules the night before and just before you go to bed.

Now, Oxy-Powder is not a laxative, so they are not addictive. What these capsules do is supply oxygen to your colon, which dissolves the hard fecal matter that has built up over time and has not wanted to come out.

Because this bottle of Oxy-Powder has 125 capsules, you can take 1 to 3 capsules during your 10-day weight-loss program.

Oxy-Powder causes your stools to become watery, since it is dissolving the hard matter in your colon. Don't be concerned that you have diarrhea like symptoms. In addition, this three day cleanse will also cause you to have watery stools, since you are on a diet of juices and fruits. This process is cleaning out your colon.

If you chose to use prune juice to clear out your colon, this procedure will be described below.

First day of colon cleanse

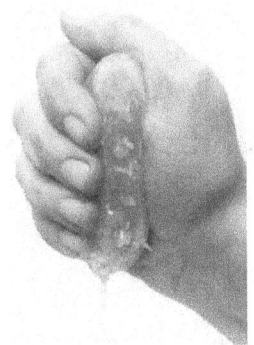

Do this cleanse on a Saturday, Sunday or any other day that you don't have to go anywhere. You may be going to the bathroom all day, and at times you need to be there quick. But, you can do this cleanse even during a work day.

This first morning, you will have a bowel movement when you wake up, because of the Oxy-Powder. After that, go do your lemon drink.

Lemon Juice Drink - Every morning when you first get up, drink a glass of slightly warm water with the juice of 1/2 lemon. This will remove mucus from your intestinal tract and detoxify your liver.

Prune Juice Colon Cleanse

If you decided to use prune juice to clean out your colon, instead of Oxy-Powder, then here is what you need to do.

However, you can also do prune juice, if you have done the Oxy-powder since the prune juice is filled with minerals and nutrients that will cleanse your body.

- About 1/2 hour after your lemon drink, take 8 oz. of prune juice.

- 10 minutes later drink another 8 oz. of prune juice

- 10 minutes later again drink another 8 oz. of prune juice

- wait 20 minutes than drink 8 oz. of apple juice

- wait 30 minutes than drink another 8 oz. of apple juice

If you haven't sped to the bathroom yet, you will, in a little while.

Now drink 8 oz. of apple juice every hour until the end of the day. You can stop drinking apple juice around 5pm. You can use different fruit juices or vegetable juices in place of apple juice, but, just make sure you drink mostly apple juice.

During the day, you can eat 1 or 2 apple in the morning and 1 in the evening.

Second Day Of The Colon Cleanse

During the second day, you can drink different kinds of juices and eat 2-6 apples. You can drink any kind of juice be it fruit or vegetable. A combination of fruit and vegetable juice is good. You can add other fruits to eat such as watermelon, melon, oranges, and strawberries.

Third Day Of The Colon Cleanse

The third day is like the second day where you can drink different kinds of juice and eat 2-6 apples or other fruit.

On this day, you can eat other fruits like mango, watermelon, cantaloupe, and pineapple. At the end of this day, you can eat a salad with a variety of vegetables.

Fourth Day Start Of Colon Cleanse

You can continue to use Oxypowder at 2 capsules every night for the rest of the month.

Now you're ready to start your weight-loss program, so let's get stated.

6: Lose Weight Using Your body cycles

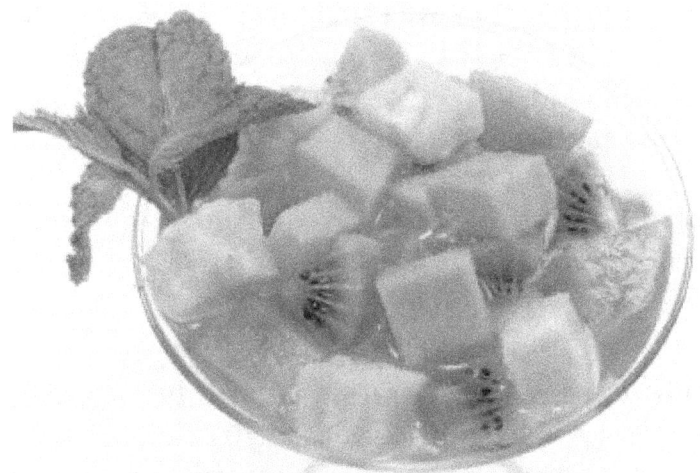

Discover Your Natural Body Cycles

You are now ready to discover the power of your body cycles. As mentioned before, using these cycles properly allow you to cleanse your body daily to keep toxins and excess fat from accumulating in your body.

Your body has natural cycles where it performs various body functions at certain times, such as digestion, detoxifying, and elimination. If you interfere with these cycles, you suppress these functions and this leads to increase weight and disease.

By learning how to assist your "Body's Natural Cycles," you will be in tune with what your body is doing to eliminate fecal matter from the colon and toxic wastes from your lymph liquid and blood.

Getting in tune with your Natural Body Cycles requires a change to the way you eat. Since all of us are addicted to the way we eat, it is, sometimes, difficult to change these habits. But, this is the best information that will give you great health and keep you at your normal weight.

Here are the 3 natural body cycles:

Cycle 1 time period: 4 am to noon

This cycle is the time where your body is eliminating toxins, acids, wastes, and derby through urine, bowel movements, and other secretions. Most people interfere with this cycle, since they are unaware of it, causing constipation, increase weight and various detrimental illnesses.

Cycle 2 time period: noon to 8 pm

This is the time when your body should be taking in food and digesting it. By eating the right kind of food, you help your digestive process in your stomach and small intestine. This is your first and second meal of the day – lunch and dinner.

Cycle 3 time period: 8 pm to 4 am

This is the time your body is absorbing and using food you have eaten from noon to 8 pm. Various organs are detoxifying and producing waste and moving it into your kidney and colon. When you wake up, this is the waste you should be getting rid, during body cycle one.

Using Your Body Cycles

Once you finish your cleanse, you are ready to start your new eating pattern. Using the Body Cycles will help you to detoxify your body daily, lose weight, keep your weight off, and improve your health.

You are ready to start practicing Body Cycle 1

This cycle is from the time you get up to noon time. During this time, you only want to eat fruits, drink juices, vegetables, and teas. This cycle helps you get rid of toxins that your body has accumulated during the night. It does this by urine and bowel movements. You can help your body by providing liquid and nutrients to help detoxify it.

Your morning breakfast will consist of a first morning drink, bowl of mixed fruits, vegetable, fruit juice, unprocessed oat cereal with fruits, or a smoothie.

Before noontime, eat fruits as snacks. Forty-five minutes before noon eat your last fruit. You can eat and drink all the fruits and juices you want up to noontime.

Fruits contain the right balance of nutrients with about 70% distilled water. Eat them without cooking them. They are easy to digest and absorb and do not stress your colon. They activate peristaltic action in your colon and help you have a bowel movement.

Morning Drink

Here are a few of the different types of drinks you should use in the morning.

When you first get up, drink one of the following drinks. Each day you can choose a different drink or you can change every week to get the benefits of the different drinks.

a. Eight oz. of water with one lemon juice – detoxifies the liver. This you can drink first. (Drink an 8 oz. glass of lemon water 15 to 20 minutes before every meal. This will help fill you up and help you to keep your portions under control. Many people mistake thirst for hunger, so staying hydrated is a good way to help regulate your appetite.)

b. Eight oz. of water with one lemon juice and 1 to 3 tablespoons of chlorophyll liquid – improves blood and detoxifies the stomach, intestines, blood, and colon.

c. A tea of ginger – improves blood circulation

d. A cup of green tea – helps to detoxify your body and is good for your cardiovascular system.

e. A glass of a mixture of 3 citrus fruits. With a hand juicer, prepare a mixture of one orange, one grapefruit, and one lemon – helps to detoxify the body and starts eliminating acids from your body. Use this drink only once or twice a week.

f. A glass of tomato juice with the juice from one lemon – provides lycopene, anti-oxidants, and builds blood - helps you to lose weight.

g. Take a glass of green drink. You can buy some super green powders that contain all kinds of nutrients and plenty of green vegetable power. Add some honey to sweeten the taste. Some of these green drinks don't taste so good.

Shower Time

After your morning drink, you can take a shower and get dressed. After you do this, you are ready for the next step.

Morning Fruit

Now you are ready to have some fruit, fruit pudding, vegetable juice, or morning shake. Vary what you eat at this point so that you can give your body a variety of nutrients that will help to promote a good bowel movement. Here are some of the best fruits to eat:

Apples   Apricots

Avocados   Bananas
Blueberries Boysenberries
Cantaloupes   Cherries
Grapes   Lemons
Nectarines   Figs and dates
Oranges   Papayas
Peaches   Pears
Persimmons   Plums
Prunes   Raspberries
Strawberries   Watermelons

Here are a few morning breakfast suggestions:

a. Slices of watermelon, cantaloupes, or any other type of melon. You can mix them together – helps to eliminate acids from your body and promotes urine. Eat these fruits together and don't mix them with other fruits. Wait 1/2 hour before eating other fruits.

b. A bowl of different fruit such as apple, mango, pineapple, strawberries, and berries. Choose those fruits on the list provided that will provide you with a lot of fiber – fiber will help you lose weight and keep your colon clean. Remember you need to eat up to 30 to 35 grams of fiber in this eating habits program.

c. A bowl of the special soup as outlined in the previous chapter. This soup you can eat anytime that you get hungry. So, you will want to take some to work in a thermos. The liquid and vegetables will help to promote a bowel movement.

d. A pudding of different fruits that you put into a blender. Add some apple juice or other juices you like, to adjust the pudding consistency. This helps to give you fiber, make your body more alkaline, and activates peristaltic action . You can put some of this pudding in a thermos and use it for snacks during the morning or afternoon break.

e. A smoothie as outline in the next chapters. Use this type of smoothie only 1 or 2 times a week – fiber and special nutrients help you to lose weight and to keep you healthy.

f. On occasion, you can eat a pouched egg or a small amount of whole oats, not the quick-cooking oats. You can use apple juice to dilute the oats and add a banana and raisins. You can do this once a week, if you like.

You can use your own ideas of how you want to eat fruits and vegetables at this time. I have just given you some ideas to start.

Avoid Heavy Morning Breakfast

Eating solid food for breakfast – eggs potatoes, rice, meat, cereal, milk, and so on, the typical breakfast, interferes with your body's elimination cycle and eventually leads to sickness and excess weight.

It takes over three hours to digest heavy and solid food. The food you should be eating in the morning should digest quickly. This helps you to activate peristaltic colon movement to create a bowel and to continue your body's detoxification and elimination process.

Acids are the main cause of most illnesses, so you want to have an alkaline body. Fruits and vegetables neutralize acids and give you an alkaline body. An alkaline body is the healthiest body condition you can have.

It takes 1 to 1 1/2 hour or so to digest fruits and fruit juices. Because of this, they help to cleanse your body of waste during the time from 4am to noontime.

Morning Snack

During your morning and afternoon break, it's time to open your thermos and have a good snack. Make sure you take your snack breaks. Use only fruits, vegetables, nuts, and soups for your snacks. These types of snacks help you to digest your food better and also activate peristaltic colon action. They give you fiber and many of the minerals you need to make your body more alkaline

Usually, morning snack time is around 10 am. At this time, you want to have the following type of snacks.

a. Eat the special soup that you have prepared and that is in your thermos.

b. Eat more fruit like apples, strawberries, or watermelon – helps reduce body acid, provides fiber, and helps you to eliminate body toxins through urine and stools.

c. Drink some leftover smoothie that you brought in a thermos.

d. Drink some juice that was mentioned in the previous chapter – helps to promote bowel movements and keep your body alkaline.

Juices To Drink

Here are the juices to drink during your break time or for your smoothies. You can drink many of the other juices listed in the other chapters. You can also make fresh juices with these fruits in a juicer. When you do, include some of the pulp in your juice to get some fiber.

FRUIT JUICE, UNSWEETENED
- Apple juice/cider
- Cranberry juice cocktail
- Cranberry juice cocktail, reduced-calorie
- Fruit juice blends, 100% juice
- Grape juice
- Grapefruit juice
- Orange juice

- Prune juice

The Second Natural Body Cycle - Lunch Time

Here is the second body cycle, and it occurs from noon to 8 pm.

Noon is the time to eat heavy food. It is this food that is going to give you the nutrients to provide your body with energy and to help it regenerate itself.

For lunch, you only want to eat enough food for your daily needs. When you eat more than what your body needs to keep it going, it will turn the excess into fat.

Here is some food that you should be eating for lunch.

a. Always eat a raw salad or raw vegetables with your main meal. Look at the list of vegetables and try to eat those that have the most fiber. But, mix them by eating some with a lot of fiber and some with low fiber. If you eat cooked vegetables, cook them for a few minutes to minimize the degradation of the fiber.

b. You can eat all the vegetables you want from the list that is called non starchy vegetables. These vegetables will not make you gain weight.

c. Your main course can be any of the meat, poultry, or fish listed in the previous chapter.

The severing size listed is not the amount you should eat. You can eat an amount to where you feel satisfied, but do not overeat. Protein can also be stored as fat, when your body does not need it. If you eat plenty during cycle 1, you will not need to eat a lot of meat at noon time. For your meals, always eat one type of meat. Do not mix your proteins. For example, don't eat beef and fish in one meal.

d. The best protein to eat is fish. Beef has been found to contribute to cardiovascular diseases. So try to minimize the use of beef, if you eat it. Or, you can just reduce the serving size of beef.

e. Try to eat only one meat and vegetables – helps to improve your digestion and reduces any stomach problems. Most people are used to eating meat potatoes or rice with vegetables. If you need rice, use a reduced amount of rice.

When you eat any animal protein, avoid eating it with non-starchy vegetables - artichokes, yams, sweet potatoes, carrots, oats, peas, potatoes, rice, wheat, winter squash and corn. These vegetables break down into sugars that coat your protein food and this causes a chemical process called glycation, which creates inflammation and lowers your immunity. In addition, this combination of protein and starches is difficult to digest and disrupts your second body cycle.

When you eat animal protein, eat it with broccoli, cabbage, cauliflower, celery, cucumber, garlic, green beans, leafy greens onions, garlic, wakame, dulse, and zucchini.

f. Don't drink any juice, water, soda, or sweet drinks with your lunch – improves your digestion. You can drink some room-temperature water to clear your throat. Drinking a cold liquid will slow down your digestion.

g. During lunch is a good time to add a dressing to your salad. This dressing should contain some fatty oils, such as olive oil, flax oil, a small of mayonnaise. You can eat some saturated fat, since the body needs it, but do it in small amounts. Don't pour it on thick.

h. Don't eat any deserts after your lunch and especially fruits – this interrupts your digestion process. Wait about an hour before eat a desert.

i. Or, you can eat only brown or red rice or other grains, with both starchy and non-starchy vegetables, with no meat.

j. It is permissible to eat beef and chicken at the same time but not chicken and eggs or beef and nuts or chicken and beans. Eat the same type of protein at the same time, but do not mix different proteins.

Eating a variety of foods at the same time leads to undigested food. Food that is partially undigested becomes acidic, which affects the health of your colon and causes constipation. When these acids are absorbed into your body, they are converted into fat and stored as toxins your body.

Eating the right combination of foods at meal time, helps you to preserve your energy for the elimination cycle and prevents you from creating spoiled food in your stomach that is converted to acid waste. It is this acid waste that results in illness and fat. This is the reason most people as they age become overweight and come down with various illnesses that terminate their lives early.

After Lunch Snack

For afternoon snacks, use the ideas given for Morning Snacks.

Notice that you can eat many foods that you cannot in other diets. When you eat foods that you like, do it in small quantities.

Learn to eat less of the foods you like and eat more

frequently. Always eat something during morning and afternoon snack time.

   a. You can use nuts or seeds as snacks but do it in moderation – gives you some of the omega-3 and -6 fatty acids.

   b. Eat some of the special soup you still have in your thermos – helps you lose weight.

   c. Drink some juice like cherry juice, prune juice, apple juice or pineapple juice.

   d. Eat some fruit from the list provided.

Dinner time

This is the time to eat carbohydrates or more protein. It is best to eat carbohydrates with vegetables and no protein. You may find this hard to do but here is what to eat at dinner time.

   a. Brown rice with cooked vegetable and or a salad. You can eat all the brown rice you want, but don't over eat. If you are not used to eating without some meat, add a small amount of meat to the rice.

   b. You can interchange your dinner type meal with your lunch meal. Concentrate your lunch meal with carbohydrates and a little meat and at dinner concentrate on protein with a little carbohydrate.

c. Eat less meat for dinner and no fish for dinner, since meat takes a long to digest. Also, fish takes longer to digest than meat.

d. You can eat some pasta, provided you eat plenty of raw vegetables. But, watch the pasta, since over eating can cause you some weight gain.

After Dinner Snacks

Try not to eat anything 2 to 3 hours before bedtime. If you need a snack, here is a starter list.

a. Fruits like pineapple, apple, and so on – helps to provide the minerals needed to neutralize body acids.

b. Here again, you can have some vegetable soup – this soup helps you from getting or staying hungry and will not cause you to gain weight.

The Third Body Cycle

The third body cycle is the assimilation cycle and is from 8pm to 4am. This is the time the food you have eaten during the day is assimilated, absorbed and distributed throughout your body through your blood. It is the time where digested food moves into the colon as chime and is stored there for elimination.

And, you should be eliminating this chime or fecal matter, when you wake up or during the morning to noon.

Food eaten during the second cycle, noon to 8 pm, and that was combined and eaten properly will digest within 3 to 4 hours, whereas food not combine properly, a meal consisting of protein and carbohydrates, will take up to 8 hours to pass through your stomach. During this time, some of your food will putrefy and ferment and become acidic. Under these conditions, you will not get many nutrients from that meal.

So, eat your last meal by 6-7 pm, so that your food digests in your stomach by the time you go to bed. After three hours later, your food will have moved into your small intestine where it is ready for assimilation.

When you go to bed three hours after your last meal, the next six hours, until 4am, your body will be absorbing the food you have eaten the previous day and moving waste into your colon.

Remember, anything you do different than what these cycles call for will disrupt them and cause them to become extended and your cycle time will be off. Just start changing your eating habits slowly and as time passes you will be doing more and more of what your body's natural cycles need.

7: Acid Alkaline Fruits Foods To Eat

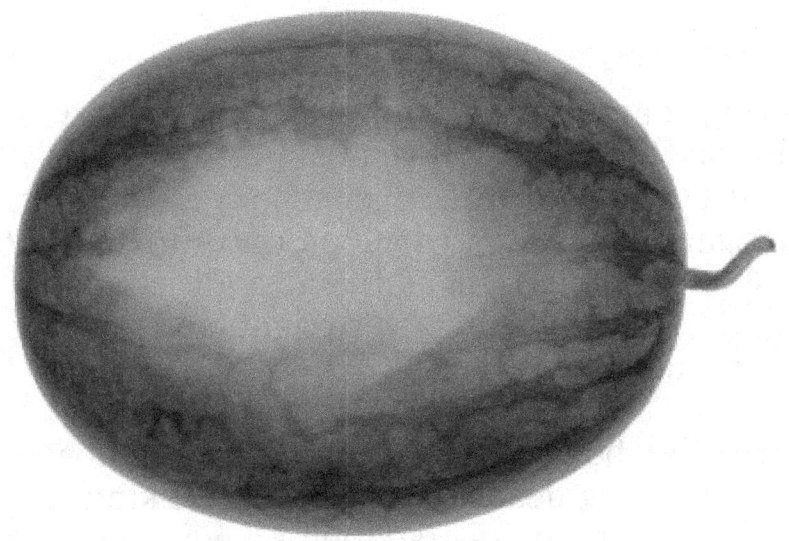

Alkaline Body

Losing weight and maintaining a healthy body go hand in hand. You cannot be healthy and be overweight. At some point in your life, you will develop a condition or illness that is related to your excess weight or to an acid body.

Of course, not being overweight doesn't mean you are healthy. To be in good health, you need to have an excellent lifestyle, and this means eating and living healthy.

When you eat natural food that gives you good health, your body will be alkaline and this condition produces better health. In this chapter, you will discover what it means to have an acid body and an alkaline body. Then you will see what foods you need to eat to have an alkaline body.

Minerals

Moving your body more toward alkalinity is what will help you lose weight. If you have an acid body, it will be hard to lose weight. An acid body attracts disease, pathogens, and water, which produces toxins that can be stored as fat. In addition, a diseased body is associated with being overweight and lacking the proper nutrition.

An alkaline body prevents your body from becoming ill and forming deadly diseases, like all kinds of joint problems, organ degradation, body pain, heart disease, or even cancer. If you are already sick, then all the chemicals inside fruits will help to revive you to better health. This is provided that your tissue damage has not gone beyond repair.

The minerals most important in changing and maintaining your body in an alkaline condition are sodium, potassium, chloride, calcium, phosphorus, magnesium, and sulphur.

Now, how your body can become alkaline might become a little confusing at first because of the terms used, but let's break this down into small parts. First, we are going to be defining some terms, so we can then start talking the same language.

Acid Binding

There are certain minerals that are called acid binding. And these are minerals we said are the most important ones in fruits - Sodium, potassium, chloride, calcium, phosphorus, and magnesium - because they are acid binding.

What acid binding means is when you eat fruits with these minerals, they will combine with acids in your body and neutralize them. These neutralized acids will be then be eliminated from your body in your urine and feces.

If not all the acid toxins are captured by acid binding matter, the remaining acids can be neutralized by body stores of alkaline minerals. If you don't have a good store of alkaline minerals, then these acids will remain in your body creating disease. But, if you do have a good store of alkaline minerals, these minerals will find acids, capture them, and bind with them. Then these acids will be moved out of your body, by your urine, stools, and breath.

So you can see the importance of getting a lot of alkaline minerals into your body. Without them, acids would not get eliminated from your body, and they would remain in your body tissue and continue their body damage.

Acid binding minerals mainly come from eating vegetables and fruits.

Alkaline Binding

Now, there are also minerals that become alkaline binding and these minerals are sulphur, chlorine, iodine, phosphorus, bromine, fluorine, copper, and silicon. It is these minerals that when digested by a cell will produce a salt that will bind with alkaline minerals. These minerals will be excreted through your urine.

When alkaline minerals are trapped by an acid salt, the alkaline mineral is removed from your body, and your body becomes more acidic. This is the condition you are trying to avoid.

Foods that are alkaline binding and remove the minerals that you need to make your body alkaline are meat, carbohydrates, some vegetables and some fruits.

Although you need to eat both foods that are acid binding or alkaline binding, you want to eat more of the acid binding foods. This will keep your body slightly alkaline.

Where do Acid Toxins Come From?

So why is the body overloaded with toxins? Why can't the liver take care of these toxins? Your liver has the function to remove acid wastes from natural food that is created by food digestion and cell metabolism. When your body encounters acid wastes, such as food enhancers, dyes, preservatives, pesticides, and the variety of additives, the liver does not know how to break them down or make them harmless.

But, your body does not give up so easily, when it knows that the liver is not able to disintegrate food additives. What it does is it instructs calcium to bind with these toxic acids and remove them from your blood stream.

Now, we have talked about acid toxins in the body that are brought in through food and the environment. But, there is another factor that creates acid in the body and that is emotions that are activated through life stresses, like work pressures, divorce, friendship problems, martial issues, and other similar situations. These emotional problems create acidic molecules that then embed themselves into your tissues just like food acids. These again can be removed with minerals.

Body Organs

All body organs function to rid the body of acid waste or toxins. Lack of acid binding food causes the deterioration of these organs. Each organ has a specific function in the elimination and neutralization of acid wastes, and it does this in conjunction with acid binding minerals.

Acid Binding Foods

Here is a list of the fruits that have the highest

alkaline minerals and the ones that you should be eating to eliminate your body's acids.

The percentage assigned to these fruits is based on fresh fruits that are organic, and that they are not cooked, canned or mixed with sugar. If they are cooked or otherwise processed in some fashion, this will reduce their effectiveness as an acid binding fruit. However, they will still be somewhat effective in acid binding.

Fruits above 50% in value are more acid binding, which means they will trap acid wastes better. You will want to eat and drink those fruits above 51%.

The fruits that are at 50% at are neutral. They are not acid binding nor alkaline binding.

Here is the list of fruits to eat and drink in the order of priority.

1. Fruits at 100% Acid Binding – Best fruits To Eat And Drink

Lemons, melons – any type, watermelon
2. Fruits at 93% Acid Binding – Great fruits To Eat And Drink

Cantaloupes, dried dates, dried figs, limes, mango, papaya
3. Fruits at 87% Acid Binding – Still Great Fruits To Eat And Drink

Kiwis, passion fruit, pineapples, raisins, umeboshi plums

4. Fruits at 80% Acid Binding – Eat And Drink These Fruits

5. Apricots, avocados, bananas, fresh dates, fresh figs, currants, gooseberries grapes, grapefruits guavas, kumquats, nectarines, pears, persimmons, quince

6. Fruits at 73% Acid Binding – Still Fruits To Eat And Drink

Apples, organs, peaches, pomegranate, raspberries, sour grapes, strawberries

7. Fruits at 67% Acid Binding – Still Neutralizes Acids, Eat And Drink This fruit

Cherries

Fruits To Concentrate On

These are the fruits you should concentrate on eating. Also, eat them every day, if possible, fresh lemon juice in the morning, watermelon during the day.

You can see which fruits give you the best acid binding effects and eating and drinking them 80% of your overall food intake will convert your body over to an Alkaline body.

8: How Fiber Helps You Get Rid of Pounds

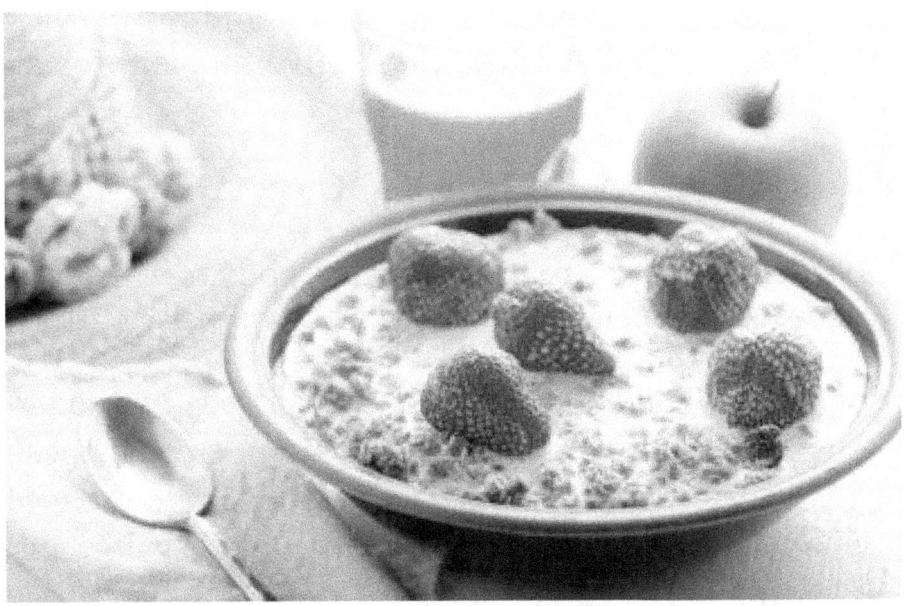

What is Fiber All About?

One of the best ways to lose weight is to use fiber. There is no way that you can lose weight and keep it off, if your weight-loss program does not contain and use fiber.

Weight loss is about controlling the amount of calories you consume and the calories you burn. Since fiber does not contain calories, you can eat all the fiber you want. But, fiber is found only in produce, so this means you can eat all the produce you want.

Fiber is also the foundation for maintain your health. If you do not eat fruits and vegetables, you will be susceptible to obesity, colon diseases, cardiovascular irregularity, constipation, varicose veins, hemorrhoids, and gout. I can go on and on, but it's not necessary. Fiber is the preventive nutrient for all disease.

Fiber Benefits You Need To Know About

Fiber has a way of regulating your body, so that you don't eat more calories than your body needs.

1. When you eat one gm. of fiber, it ties up 8 or so calories in your digestive system, so that these calories don't get into your blood stream. These 8 calories of food are routed to your colon and expelled in your stools.

2. **Fiber is a food digestive suppressant.**

   a. If you eat 37 gm. of fiber every day, you will excrete 8 x 37 calories in your stools. This amounts to 297 calories that don't get absorbed into your body. If you don't eat fiber during the day, you will absorb an additional 297 calories.

3. When the food you eat passes your stomach and goes into your small intestine, a chemical is released called Cholecystokinin. This chemical signals your gallbladder and pancreas to release

bile and digestive enzymes to digest the food in your small intestine. Once digested, this food is absorbed through the intestine walls and moves into your blood.

In clinical studies, it was found that the more Cholecystokinin, CCK, in the small intestine the more a person would feel full and would stop eating. When you eat fiber, more CCK is released than when you eat foods that do not contain fiber. **Fiber helps to make you feel full and satisfied** quicker than when you eat non-fiber food.

4. Fiber in your stomach has the benefit of reducing the speed at which carbohydrates are converted into sugar and released into the small intestine. Fiber can increase insulin sensitivity. If you have diabetes, fiber is the nutrient to use to control your sugar blood level.

Cooking fruits and vegetables that have insoluble fiber weaken their strength and benefits. Cook vegetables only with a little water and for a few minutes until they are slightly soft.

Types Of Fiber

There are two types of fiber – soluble and insoluble. You need both to maintain health and lose weight.

Soluble Fiber

Soluble Fiber become gummy and viscous after it dissolves in water.

Soluble fiber can slow down digestion in the small intestine and prevent simple sugars from entering the bloodstream right away.

Because it absorbs water, soluble fiber softens and gives weight to fecal matter, and this makes fecal matter easier to pass through your colon.

Soluble fiber consists of pectin, gum, and mucilage. Pectin is found in carrots, apples, beets, cabbage, citrus fruits, and bananas. Gums and mucilage are found in oat bran, sesame seeds, oats, oatmeal, legumes, guar gum, and arabic gum
Benefits of soluble fiber:

- reduces the risk of heart disease

- reduces the risk of gallstones

- helps to remove toxic heavy metals and toxins from your colon

- helps to prevent the toxic condition call appendicitis

- helps to prevent hemorrhoids and fissures

- lowers cholesterol

- lowers absorption of fats in the intestines

- helps prevent the overgrowth of bad bacteria in your colon.

Insoluble Fiber

Insoluble fiber does not dissolve in water and consists of cellulose, hemi cellulose, and lignin. This type of fiber is extremely beneficial for your health. Because your body's enzymes cannot break down this fiber, like it does food, it remains in tack as it travels through your intestines and colon.
Insoluble fiber helps the fecal matter travel faster through the small intestine and your colon.

It provides the bulk to your fecal matter. It makes your stools larger, softer, and stimulates peristaltic movement as it touches your colon walls.

Insoluble fiber, like soluble fiber, slows down digestion. It also slows down absorption of protein, starch and fat and can inhibit the action of digestive enzymes.

Insoluble fibers are found in vegetables, wheat, and wheat bran. This type of fiber is considered an anti-carcinogen and a digestive aid. It is credited with preventing colon cancer and many other colon diseases.

Cellulose – Insoluble Fiber

Cellulose is a nondigestible carbohydrate which is found in the skins of fruits and vegetables – peas, green beans, carrots, broccoli, beets, brazil nuts, and lima beans.

Cellulose helps to remove cancer-causing toxins from your colon walls. It helps to prevent constipation, colitis, varicose veins, and hemorrhoids.

Hemi-cellulose is found in cabbage, peppers, green vegetables, and beets. The benefits of this fiber are:

- absorbs water in your colon and makes your stools softer
- aids in weight loss
- prevents constipation
- decreases the chances of colon cancer
- controls the carcinogens in the intestinal tract

Lignin – Insoluble Fiber

Lignin is also an insoluble fiber. It is found carrots, peas, tomatoes, bran, and green beans.

Fiber is involved in your digestion and can,

- improve nutrient absorption
- increase stool weight
- increase good bacterial activities in intestines
- improve composition of the fecal matter

- Make fecal matter travel faster and easier out the colon
- absorb water to create bulk in the fecal matter
- absorb cholesterol and move it out the rectum
- sweep clean your colon walls and remove toxins, waste,
- debris and other contaminates and moves them out your colon.
- provide food for the good bacteria

Seaweed fiber

Agar and alginate come from seaweed and are indigestible. They are used in gelatinous foods to make desserts. Alginate is especially useful since it can bind to harmful metals such as lead, arsenic, mercury, and cadmium and move them out of your body through your stools.

Actions To Take From This Chapter

1. Start eating more fiber in your diet. Add it gradually every day or week.

2. Eat fiber with each meal. For breakfast eat fruits and with meals eat fresh and slightly cooked vegetables.

3. Eat a variety of fruits and vegetables. Use the idea of eating a variety of different color produce. 6:For every 3,500 calories you don't eat or take off your diet, you will lose 1 pound over a certain time period.

4. Drink at least 4-6 glasses of water when adding more fiber to your diet to avoid any side effects.

9: How Juices Help You Lose Pounds

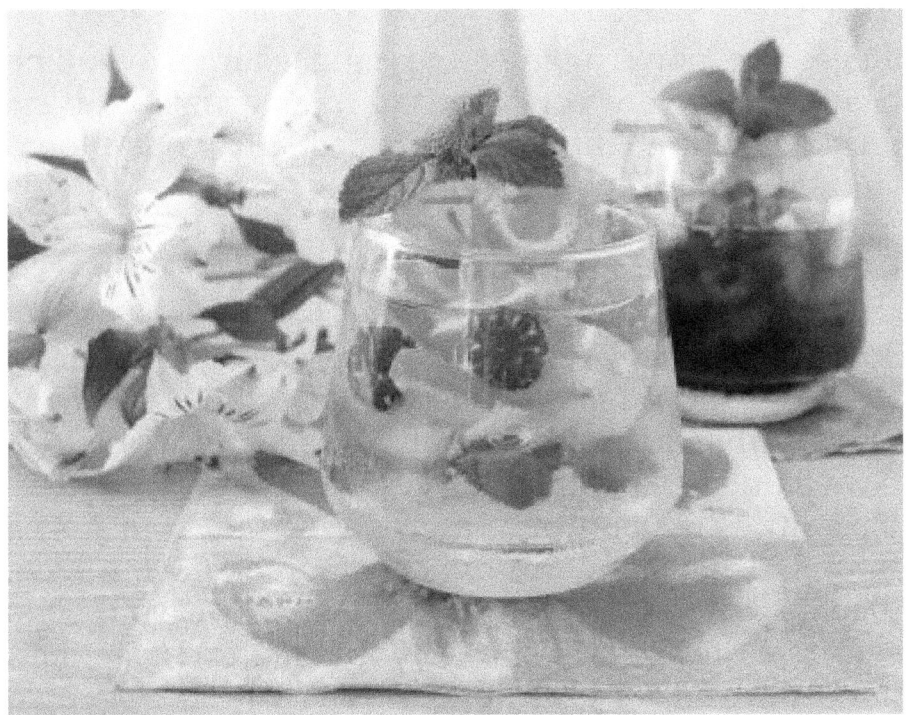

Juices for Health

Here are some of the fruits that I listed in the previous lesson. I give you information on some of the best fruit to eat.

Use them between meals, before meals, in some cases, or just two hours before bedtime. You can also drink the juices that are listed in the previous lesson that are not listed here. The important thing is you can target certain juices for specific illness, or use them as a general body tonic. Use a variety of juices to get the benefit of the different nutrients that these fruit juices have.

Juices are powerful remedies and sources of quick health. They are concentrated in nutrients and are quickly, within minutes, absorbed into your blood, since they require little or no digestion. For this reason, you can use them to rebuild, cleanse, and detoxify your body quickly and easily.

Juices can help you prevent, retard, or cure illness. However, they must be used properly and at the right times. In some cases, use of juices as a therapy can have side effects, but when used in moderation they have little side effects. There are certain fruit juices that are high in natural sugars, so if you have diabetes, it is best to avoid them. If you have sensitive throats or respiratory issue, then you should not use citrus juices. And, there are also some people that are allergic to specific fruits.

All diseases respond to specific fruit juices because they correct and rebalance the heat or cold in the body. They remove and neutralize toxins. So, use them when you have a fever or when you have a cold.

It is always best to juice those fruits that are grown locally. The nutrients supplied by these fruits are related to the surrounding climate and environment and provide you with the nutrients that you need. It is ok to drink exotic juices like mango, pineapple, guava, and other tropical juices, but these should be kept to around 20% of the juices you drink.

At times, juices can pull out too many toxins from your body, if you are too toxic, causing you to feel sick and uneasy. Some people get an upset stomach, if they drink juices the first thing in the morning.

Juice side effects can range from headaches to rashes or pain. Side effects will subside as you drink the juices and continue to detoxify your body.

Fresh juices are easy to create with a juicer and give you the pleasure of knowing you are giving your body the nutrients it needs. They give you a quick lift because of the nutrients and the natural sugar they contain. Once in your mouth, nutrients and sugar immediately enter your blood and are delivered soon after into your cells. This is why they are good for people who are recovering from an illness or are trying to re-develop good health.

Always use fresh juice when possible. One glass of juice can count as more than one serving of fruit. Bottled juice no longer has the pH that fresh juice has and loses a slight amount of its pH value. This means bottled juice may be acidic instead of alkaline.

However, when certain juices are not available fresh, it is always best to use bottled or packaged juice to preserve your health.

Avoid buying juices in cans, aluminum containers, and plastic bottles. These juices have been highly processed and tend to have reduced nutritional value.

Using Juices

Once you create your juice, you should drink it right away. If you plan to take it to work, add a teaspoon of vitamin C powder or the juice of half lemon to act as a preservative. Store the thermos in the refrigerator, if possible. If not possible, then you should drink the juice with a couple of hours.

The amount of juice that you should use is dependent on many items. For weight loss, you want to drink those juices that contain more fiber. Normally, juicing removes most of the fiber, except some of the more expensive juicers maintain the fiber in the juice. Drinking juices will help you lose weight. The reason is that juices help you remove acid and waste from your body. Acid and waste are sometimes converted over to fat. Fresh juices give you the fiber factor that you need for losing weight.

Fruits to Use

In one of the chapters is a list of which fruits are best for turning an acid body to an alkaline body. These are the fruits that you should use and eat. Keep in mind that one juice may help one person for a particular condition and for another it may not help at all. But, in general, juices are a powerful way to recover health.

Lemons

Citrus fruits such as lemons, limes, oranges and grapefruits have chemicals that reduce your insulin levels and promoting losing weight.

Before juicing lemons, roll then on a table top to get them slightly soft. Lemons added to other juices give them additional flavor or soften their sweetness or saltiness. Lemons are antiseptic and act as a powerful cleanser for the entire body. You can take a small sip of lemon juice before a meal to cleanse your stomach and the small intestine.

Drinking lemon juice with warm water in the morning is useful in restoring chemical balance in your body. It restores the positive and negative chemical ions in your body to a more natural state. In addition, it helps the liver create many different digestive enzymes. This results in you digesting your food better and gives you an increase in energy.

Since lemon juice, just like other citrus juices, contain a high level of minerals and potassium they are especially good to drink, without sugar, during heavy work, sports, workouts, or competitive sports.

You can mix the juices of lemon, lime, oranges, and pineapple. They all have a cleansing effect upon your body. They purge and eliminate wastes from your body. You can reduce the effects of diseases such as heart, arthritis, diabetes, high blood pressure, cancer, and many other degenerative diseases by using these 4 juices together or singly. These juices will also help you lose weight.

Lime

Lime has as a similar nutritional value as oranges, but less. Lime is an excellent juice to use to recover health. But, it should be used in moderate amounts. Mixed with lemon juice, it creates a powerful healing juice. It acts as a general tonic for the whole body by energizing, restoring, and rejuvenating. It flushes out toxins and wastes from your body and re-energizes your organs.

When you wake up in the morning, put 6 oz. of distilled water into a blender, slightly warm is better but room temperature is ok. Press out the juice from one lemon and one lime and put the juice and meat into the blender, then spike with a touch of cayenne pepper. Blend for 1 minute, and drink this powerful healing juice.

Oranges

Never keep oranges in the refrigerator, since they lose their nutritional value. Squeeze your oranges in a manual orange press to get the most juice.

Oranges improve the skin complexion, assist in constipation, act as a mild laxative, remove toxins and waste from the body, act as a diuretic and improve your vision.

A glass of orange juice in the morning will activate your digestion, improve your health, and give you a feeling of well-being. Drinking a small amount after meals improves your digestion. It can be used in low amounts by diabetics.

Papayas

Papaya juice is a highly curative fruit, and its juice gives a powerful punch for health. It keeps arteries soft and flexible, preventing the deposition of cholesterol. Its digestive enzyme, pepsin, destroys the outer layer of germs, including the TB bacteria. It reduces the risk of high blood pressure, heart attacks, and improves the circulation of blood, improves liver function, restores peristaltic intestinal action, and improves vision.

Mango Juice

Mango is another health winner. Its juices help to build muscles and to strengthen tissue. It is an excellent heart and brain tonic. It is useful in constipation, digestive issues, reducing phlegm and acidity. It can expel worms, acts as an aphrodisiac, and blood rejuvenator and purifier.

Mix one part milk with two parts mango juice or puree and four parts water. You can use another juice instead of milk, since milk causes mucus.

Apples

Because apples have a high mineral content, they are especially good for your skin, hair and fingernails. Apples that are good for juices are Granny Smith, Braeburn, Egremont Russet, and Discovery. You can also juice Gala apples. If they are firm and crisp, they provide good juice. When buying apple juice, purchase the juice that is cloudy and not clear. This type of juice has more fiber and nutrients and contains a good amount of the fiber pectin.

Apple juice serves as a good base, when mixed with other juices and especially with vegetables. Most of the vitamins lie in the skin of the apple, so it is best to juice apples without peeling.

This is one of the fruits that can be used in many ways, and you still get it nutritional value. You can eat it raw, cooked, baked, juiced, jammed, or pickled.

Grape Juice

Add grape juice to other juices like apple to give it a different flavor. When juicing apples, juice a few handfuls of grapes, also. Grapes have a high content of natural sugar and can give you a quick energy lift. They contain a high level of minerals and have B vitamins. You can drink this juice from bottles, since it has a short season. In a bottle, you can drink it any time. Use the darker grape drinks, because of their high anti-oxidant nutrients.

Grapes help to regulate and increase your metabolism. A low metabolism will cause you to gain weight, and a high metabolism will help you burn food quicker.

Cherries

Fresh cherry juice is a powerful body alkalizer and reduces the acidity in your blood and tissues. It is an excellent remedy to reduce and eliminate gout pain. Gout is an excess of acid in the joints and tissue and results from eating too much protein. Drinking this juice between meals will help activate peristaltic bowel action, which can help to keep you regular.

Melons, Cantaloupes

All melons create super juices filled with the best nutrient your body can have. They are at the top of the list for making your body more alkaline. They are good for your skin and provide your nerves with the right nutrients. Melons have a cooling effect on the body and improve your digestion.

Watermelon

Watermelon juice is one of the best juices you can drink and can be obtained by simply eat raw watermelon, since it is 98% distilled water. Its use helps cleanse the kidney and bladder, since it is a diuretic – removes excess fluids from the body. You can chew on the seeds as you eat watermelon to get the extra zinc and vitamin E.

Watermelon juice tones your body, prevents heat

stroke, normalizes high blood pressure, and strengthens your heart and brain. It improves digestion, calms the nerves, and is a mild laxative.

Eat watermelon in the morning. Its juice will help you remove the nightly accumulated toxins through your urine. This will help you restore kidney function.

Pineapple Juice

Pineapple juice is another excellent juice to use frequently. Its high potassium helps to keep your nerve transmissions active. Its health value comes from its enzyme bromelain. Bromelain helps keep your body fluids balanced and neutral; It moves an acid or alkaline body to neutral.

When making pineapple juice, do not juice the center core, since it contains some harmful chemicals. You can drink pineapple juice just before a meal as an appetizer. You can also drink it 10 – 15 minutes after a meal. It helps rejuvenate and cleanse your body. It also acts as a laxative, so it helps to reduce constipation.

It is a juice and fruit to be avoided by pregnant women or women trying to get pregnant, since it contracts the uterus.

Pomegranate

Pomegranate juice controls bile and phlegm,

increases hemoglobin and purifies blood, improves appetite, and settles upset stomachs. It restores and sharpens memory, and is effective in urinary issues. It is helpful in many diseases, since it neutralizes body acids.

Strawberries

Strawberries and blueberries are very high in fiber and help you burn fat faster. By eating one cup either berry you can get up to 3.3 grams of fiber.

10: How To Using Fiber foods To Lose Weight

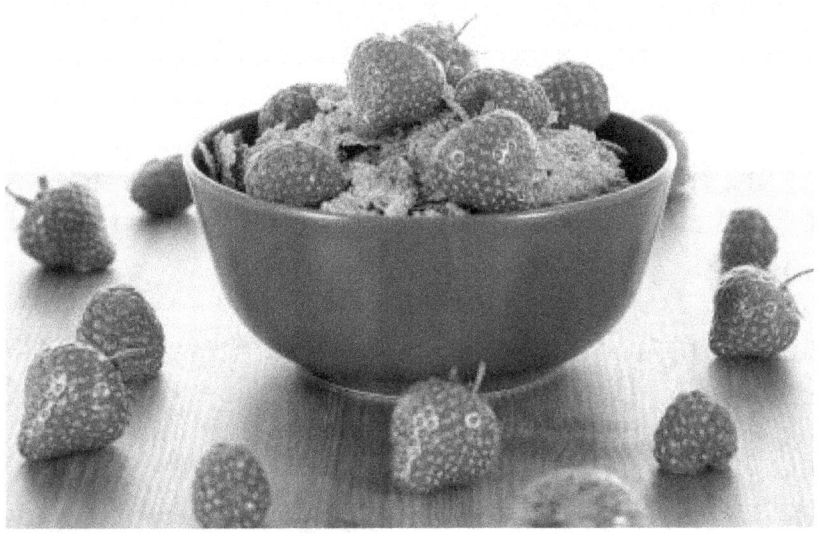

Fiber for Weight Loss

In the previous chapter, you learned that you can't lose weight without including fiber in your diet. This idea is so important that more details on using fiber are given in this chapter.

How Much Fiber Should You Eat

The amount of fiber you want to eat, eventually, is between 30 to 45 gm. The more you eat the better. Most likely, you are not eating, even, 15 gm. So, you will have to work up to eat more fiber, and you want to do it slowly. Don't all of a sudden boost your fiber level to double what you eat.

How To Add Fiber To Your Diet

Increase the fiber you eat gradually by day or by week. If you eat two fruits a day, then increase it to three per day. And, the next week increase it to four per day and the same goes for vegetables.

If you cook all your vegetables, start reducing the cooking time so that they are just Turing tender and show up slightly greener. Don't cook them until they are wilted.

Start eating more uncooked vegetables and eat them as salads. Use a natural salad dressing such as Braggs or create your own.

Side Effects of Fiber

Most fiber side effects come from eating too much fiber or eating more than you are used to. These side effects include:

1. Gas and bloating

2. Constipation

3. Stomach pain

To avoid these conditions drink more water. Make sure you are drinking 4-6 glasses of water every day and more if the fiber you eat is causing side effects.

If you are drinking morning herbal teas, fresh juices

throughout the day, or eating fruits and vegetables, all these have water and count towards your daily water total. Products like soda, sugar drinks, and any liquid with sugar do not count as water.

Fruit and Fiber

Here is a list of fruits that give you the most fiber. Try to get up to 30 to 35 grams of fiber every day. If you are short on fiber for the day look at this list of fruits and eat the ones that give you more fiber. Also, notice the fruit serving, and if you want more fiber double the serving.

FRUIT LIST Fiber	Fruit	Serving
Apple, unpeeled, small	1 (4 oz.)	4
Applesauce, unsweetened	cup	1
Apples, dried	4 rings	2
Apricots, fresh	4 whole	1
Apricots, dried	8 halves	4
Apricots, canned	½ cup	1
Banana, small	1 (4 oz.)	1
Blackberries	¾ cup	5
Blueberries	¾ cup	5
Cantaloupe, small	1 cup cubes	2
Cherries, fresh	12	2
Cherries, sweet, canned	½ cup	1
Dates	3	2-3
Figs, dried	2	2
Fruit cocktail	½ cup	1
Grapefruit, large	½	1

Grapes	17	1
Honeydew melon	1 slice	1
Kiwi	1	3
Mandarin oranges, canned	¾ cup	1
Mango, small	½ cup	1
Nectarine, small	1	2
Orange, small	1 (6 ½ oz.)	3
Papaya	½ fruit	3
Peach, fresh	1	2
Peaches, canned	½ cup	1
Pear, large, fresh	½ (4 oz.)	4
Pears, canned	½ cup	1
Pineapple, fresh	¾ cup	1
Pineapple, canned	½ cup	1
Plums, small	2	2
Raisins	2 tbsp.	1
Raspberries	1 cup	8
Strawberries	1 ¼ cup	4
Tangerines, small	2	2
Watermelon	1 ¼ cup	1

11: Weight Loss Metabolic Accelerators To Use

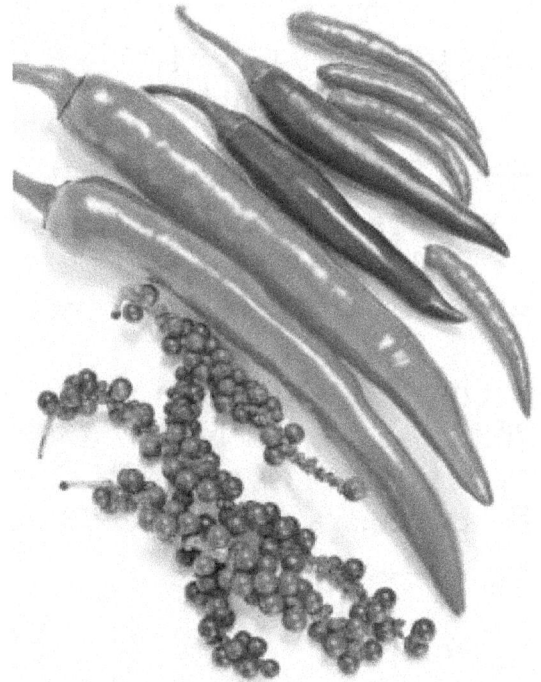

How Your Metabolism Works

Your metabolism, how fast your cells burn what you eat, and that amount of calories you eat will determine how much fat you store, and how much you will weight.

If your cells burn your nutrients fast, and you control your calorie intake to the level below what your body needs, you will lose weight quickly. If you have a fast metabolism, this is a plus for losing weight. If you have a slow metabolism, your cells will take longer to burn the nutrients you eat and your will lose weight slower.

You can also gain weight with a fast metabolism, if you eat more food that your body needs to function. How much weight you gain depends on how many calories you eat over what you need.

If your cells burn nutrients slowly and you eat more calories than you need, you will gain weight fast.

How To Increase Your Metabolism

There are certain things that you can do to increase your metabolism. This will help you greatly as you progress in your weight-loss program. Here are some of the metabolic accelerators you need to use to assist you in losing weight.

- Eat spice foods
- Protein
- Eat broccoli
- Green Tea
- Increase your immune system
- A colon and body cleanse to eliminate body toxin
- Maintain two bowel movements per day

- Make your body more alkaline
- Eat 4 to 5 small meals per day instead of 3 per day
- Drink more water than you normally do
- Sleep 8+ hours per day
- Stress
- Do muscle strengthen
- Do aerobics

Eat Spice Foods

Eating hot peppers will increase your metabolism temporarily by around 8%, which is not a whole lot, but combined with other boosters it becomes significant.

Studies have shown that by eating chilies, black pepper, or ginger, your appetite is slightly suppressed. You can try this by eating a spicy appetizer or a spicy meal.

During this program, try to eat more spicy meals. Spicy food increases your body temperature. Your body will then burn calories to bring your temperature back to normal. In addition spicy food increases your ability to burn fat.

Spicy meals, also, help to detoxify you by causing your eyes and nose to run. Also, mucus is created inside your body and is eliminated through your lymph liquid.

Lean-Protein Foods

Eating lean beef, chicken, turkey gives you the protein that you need to help you build your muscles and lose fat. In a meal, it makes you feel full and gives you energy. It increases your metabolism, which helps you lose weight. Eating a good amount of protein will help you in this program to lose weight.

Broccoli

Broccoli is a vegetable that can help you boost your metabolism. So add this vegetable to your daily diet. It is key keeping your immune system strong, and you need this to lose weight.

Green Tea

Drink the green tea that has caffeine, since caffeine increases your heart rate, causing an increase in your metabolism.

Green tea will also stimulate your fatty acids, which prevents them from being stored.

Drink one to two cups per day of green tea. Drink one cup in the morning and one in the afternoon.

Immune system

Maintaining a strong immune system, when you are

on a weight-loss program, will prevent you from getting sick. In most cases, when you lose some of your fat, your immune system improves. This occurs because fat activates hormones that suppress your immune system. These are the foods that improve your immune system.

- Oranges

- Kale

- Yogurt with Probiotics

- Garlic

- Herbal tea with honey

- Chicken soup provides acetylcysteine

- Beef to provide zinc

- Sweet potatoes, for beta-carotene

- Mushrooms - Shiitake, maitake, and reishi

- Vegetables, fruits, nuts, and seeds

Body Cleanse

Doing an initial colon and body cleanse will help you eliminate some body toxins. This reduces your weight and improves your immune system. By using the body cycles in this book, you can implement a daily detox process, which helps you eliminate toxins every day.

You can help your daily detox by drinking the following herbal tea every day.

- Dandelion

- Milk thistle

- Oregon grape root

Buy an ounce of each herb. Mix them all together. Add one teaspoon of this mixture into hot water to make a tea. Add a touch of honey to sweeten it.

Bowel Movements

If you have two bowel movements per day, you can minimize toxins from getting into your blood. The longer fecal matter remains in your colon, more toxins will move into your blood. The fewer toxins your body has the better your metabolism will work.

Drink more water than you normally do to increase your bowel movements and to flush out toxins that are being released, as you go through this weight-loss program.

Alkaline Body

Make your body more alkaline, so that your body functions better. The fewer diseases you have the sooner you will reach your normal weight.

Sleep

Getting 8 hours plus of sleep will improve your metabolism.

Stress

Reducing the stress on your liver is important in your weight-loss program. The liver is responsible for metabolizing fat. Liver stressors reduce your metabolism. To help your liver with fat metabolism, reduce the calories you eat by eliminating sugar trans fats, soda, caffeine, artificial sweeteners, and too many carbohydrates.

Exercise

By doing your exercises using the PACE method, you will help to activate your metabolism. This type of exercise will keep your improved metabolism working for you during the day and night.

12: Supplement That Can Help You Lose Pounds

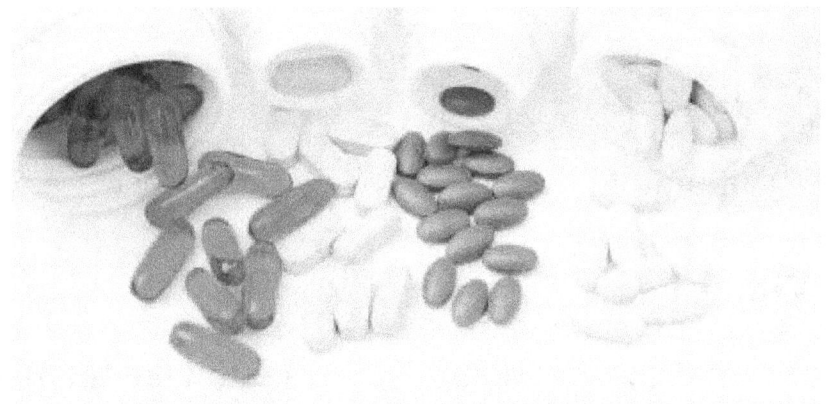

Supplement You Need

Here is a list of weight-loss supplements that can help you lose your weight. Each supplement has a different action on your body, and as you read what they can do, you can choose the right supplement for yourself.

You don't need to use all the supplements listed here, but I recommend that you use 3 to 4 of them. When you finish one bottle choose a new supplement.

Always take your supplements with meals. If you are using medication, it is best to ask your doctor about any interaction between a supplement and the drug you are using.

- B vitamins
- Banaba
- Calcium magnesium potassium
- Digestive enzymes
- FOS
- Green tea
- Minerals
- Omega 3
- Vitamin E

B Vitamins

If you want to lose weight, you need to take the B-50 or B-100 vitamins. The B-100 is a multi-vitamin supplement that contains all the B's that you need.

The B's are necessary for **proper cell metabolism,** and they increase your energy level. You will find the B-vitamins in eggs, fish, meats legumes, gains, dairy, and to some extent in leafy green vegetables.

Take one tablet per day or follow the bottle's direction.

Your body will only use the amount of B-vitamins it needs and will excrete the rest. If you like, you can start with the B-50's, which gives you 50 mg of these vitamins. When you take the B vitamins, your urine will become more yellow, which indicates you are eliminating the excess B-vitamins.

Banaba

Banaba is an herb found in the Philippines that you can use as a tea to lose weight. It has been used to treat high blood pressure, diabetes, and digestive issues.

It has been shown to stop the formation of fat cells. There are no known side effects, except that it does lower blood pressure and this could be a problem, if you are already dealing with low blood pressure.

Here's how to use it.
- 1 tea bag of Banana tea

  1 short stalk of lemon grass

  1 calamansi or lemon juice

  a bit of raw honey or stevia leaf

Magnesium-Calcium-Vitamin D

Use a supplement which contains magnesium, calcium, and vitamin D. Magnesium will give your metabolism a boost. Vitamin D is necessary for magnesium and calcium absorption.

You can increase your magnesium with the following foods: Green leafy vegetables of all kinds, nuts, whole grain cereals, oats, lentil and legumes.

Digestive Enzymes

Your blood needs good nutrition and it gets it when you properly digest your food and absorb it through your small and large intestine. By the time you are 30 years your digestive abilities has decreased considerably. To improve your digestion you need to take digestive enzymes at the start or after each meal.

Use a broadband digestive enzyme that contains amylase, protease, and lipase. If you are over 60 start testing to see if you need Betaine HCL. The amount and strength of your stomach acid, HCL, decreases as you age and your ability to digest proteins and fats decreases. Without a good amount of HCL which has a pH of 1.5-3, you cannot properly process protein and process calcium, B12, and iron. Even more important, lack of HCL limits the destruction of bad bacteria and micro-organisms - Salmonella, E.coli , and C. difficile - you eat.

Fructooligosaccharides (FOS)

FOS is a complex carbohydrate found in some fruits, grains, and herbs. It serves as food for the good bacteria found in your colon, which helps keep them strong, so they can strengthen, stabilize, and clean your colon. They also help you to absorb more calcium and magnesium.

The foods that contain FOS are onions, leeks, garlic, asparagus, burdock, and artichokes.

Keeping your colon functioning like it should, is a key to maintaining and losing weight. It is best to take an FOS supplement of 3000 mg with meals every day.

Iron

Iron is in the center of the hemoglobin blood cell. It is needed to make the hemoglobin cell. When you are low in iron, you will not form the required hemoglobin your body needs, and your metabolism will suffer. This condition is called anemia.

The oxygen needed for your cells to burn calories is provided by your hemoglobin.

You should not take iron pills, unless you are under a doctor's care. But, if you have had laboratory tests indicating you have anemia, you can eat the foods that will provide you more iron.

In fact, in this program it is recommended that you increase your iron, by eating those foods that give you more iron.

Men and older women need 8 mg. per day of iron and women up to 50 years need 18 mg. per day.

Some good food sources of iron are:

Meat, poultry, turkey, clams, and oysters

Chard   Romaine Lettuce Beef
Tenderloin

Spinach	Blackstrap Molasses	Lentils
Thyme	Shiitake Mushrooms	Brussels sprouts
Turmeric	Tofu	Asparagus
Dried Beans	Mustard Greens	Venison
Turnip Green	Garbanzo beans	String beans
Broccoli	Leeks	Kelp

Omega-3

Using a good source of omega-3, such as fish oil supplements or eating fish, is essential for your body to function like it should. Without the right amount of omega-3, omega-6, or omega-9, your body will deteriorate with disease.

The omega fatty acids will help you eliminate fat, by encouraging the releasing and using your bad fatty acids, like triglycerides.

Vitamin C

Always take vitamin C with your meals. Vitamin C is important in weight loss since it improves your immune system. You need a strong immune system so that it can neutralize and eliminate toxins, which can end up in fat cells.

This vitamin is tied to the absorption of calcium, which necessary for creating an alkaline body. You will find vitamin C in tomatoes, peppers, citrus, green vegetables and broccoli.

You should supplement with 3000 to 6000 mg of vitamin C spread out during the day.

Vitamin D

If you lack vitamin D, your weight-loss program will suffer. Clinical studies have shown that some people lose more fat, when they take more vitamin D.

You should be using from 3000 to 6000 IU of vitamin D. Some people take up to 10,000, but you need to take vitamin K when you do this.

Vitamin E

Aside from being a super antioxidant that neutralizes free radicals, vitamin E assists your body in maintaining good metabolism. You can get vitamin E in, wheat germ oil, vegetable oil, avocados, nuts, seeds leafy/green vegetables and whole grains.

13: How To Use Smoothies For Weight Loss

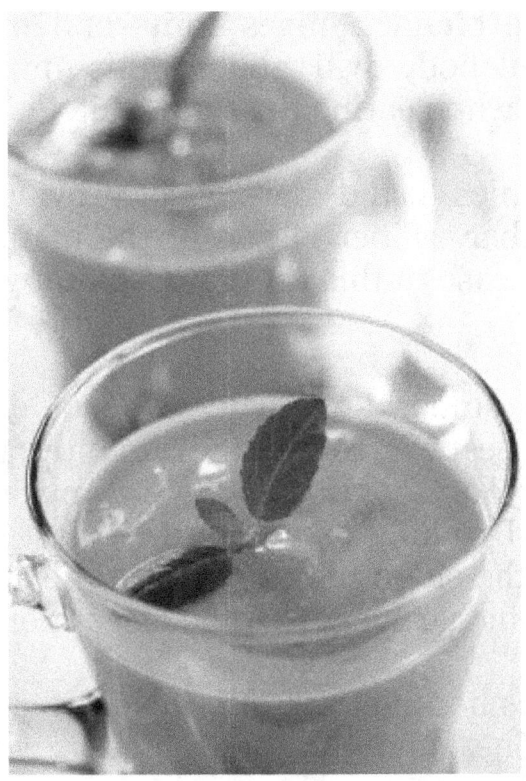

Creating Health Smoothies

Fruit smoothies provide you a different way to eat fruits and drink their juices. Smoothies mixed with other power ingredients and nutrients can serve to give you better health and help you lose weight. Smoothies can be used to build, cleanse, and heal your body.

In cases where you are depleted of various vitamins and minerals, smoothies are a way to bring these nutrients quickly into your body. When you follow the Body Cycles, smoothies have a place as part of your morning breakfast.

Because the blender mixes fruits and juices into a liquid, your body will absorb this mixture much faster, then when eating the solid fruit.

The smoothies listed here also provide you with plenty of fiber. Fiber is one of the main foods you want to increase in this program, so that you can lose weight.

Drink your smoothie slowly. Do not drink it like water. The best way to drink it is to move the mixture around in your mouth so saliva is mixed with the smoothie. Drinking a smoothie too fast can lead to gas (air in the smoothie) to form in the stomach and intestine, which can cause some discomfort.

Once your smoothie is made, drink it within a few minutes. The smoothie ingredients will start to oxidize and decay quickly as it has air mixed in from the blending process. If you fill a thermos to the top, you can use the smoothie for later, but it is always best to add a teaspoon or more of powdered vitamin C to act as a preservative.

Use fresh fruit when possible. Fresh juices will provide you with a mixture that will add more minerals to your body and thereby making your body's pH more alkaline.

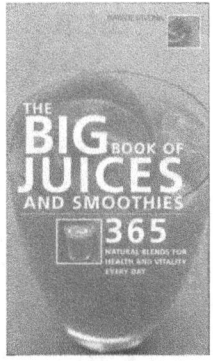

In her book, The Big Book of Juices and Smoothies, 2003, Natalie Savona, gives some hints on storing your smoothie. "there really is no such thing as storing a juice or smoothie – you can't beat drinking them the moment you've made them.

However, you may like to take them out to work or on a picnic. In that case, the best way to store them is to put a teaspoon of vitamin C powder or a squeeze of lemon juice in the bottom of the jug attached to the juicer. The vitamin C acts as an antioxidant, preventing the juice from turning brown. The same goes for smoothies. Also, keep the drinks covered and cool – in a sealed container in the refrigerator, or in a thermos flask"

Smoothie Base

Here is how you build a smoothie that can help you lose weight and give you health benefits. The smoothie base is a liquid slurry that can be used to add more ingredients.

The liquid base can be made from various fresh juices or rice, oat, or almond milks. I stay away from milk since milk creates mucus along the gastrointestinal lining and contains saturated fat. Under a maintenance diet, you can add small amounts of milk to what you eat.

Choose and mix any of the following liquid and pour them into a blender.

Juices – apple, pineapple, orange, tangerine, lemon
Milks – rice dream, oat milk, almond milk.

You can use a combination of 40% rice dream, 40% almond milk, and 20% apple juice. You can use any combination you like. For losing weight, for the first 10 days, use 80% apple juice and 20% of the other types of juices or milk.

Banana Base

Next, I always put in a banana. This gives the liquid a bit more thickness. Also, bananas are high in potassium and other minerals. Use bananas that are not overripe since they have too much sugar. Do not use under ripe bananas, since they will create acid in your body. Other under ripe fruits also create body acids.

Main Ingredients

Next I choose a fruit that will be the main ingredient so you can say you are making a strawberry smoothie or a blueberry smoothie. If you have fresh organic fruit, then this is the best way to create your smoothie. You can freeze fruits during its season, so you can have some of this fruit a bit long than its seasonal run. Choose from fruits that are in season.

- Avocado (use sparingly)

- Cantaloupe, watermelon

- Peach, mango, papaya, guava

- Pineapple, apricots, apples

- Strawberries, blueberries, raspberries

- Figs dried prunes, peaches, apricots, figs

More Nutrients to Add

Once you have your basic smoothie, you can add other nutrients that will provide you with additional fiber, oil, vitamins, minerals and many other nutrients.

Here is a shortlist of some of the ingredients you can add to your smoothies. Add only 2-3 other ingredients so the tastes don't get to complex or unusual.

- Almonds (grind to a powder with a coffee grinder)

- Beet Juice powder

- Capra mineral whey

- Chia Seeds

- ROI water ice cubes

- Edible dairy whey

- Fig Juice syrup

- Flaxseed and flax seed oil

- Honey, rice syrup

- Lecithin granules

- Powder vitamin C

- Raisins

- Rice or oat bran

- Sesame seeds

- Sunflower seeds, pumpkin seeds

- Wheat germ

A nice powder to add to your smoothie is called Ruby Reds. It adds a powerful punch to your smoothies, since it contains the powder of 35 fruit powders. This gives your smoothie a boost of vitamins, minerals, probiotics, antioxidants, photonutrients, and digestive enzymes. It's an excellent blend, and you can use with each smoothie.

Make sure you add a tablespoon or more of lecithin granules. This helps to keep your arteries clean and blood thinner. Lecithin also has choline, which helps to create acetylcholine, a neurotransmitter for your brain. Lecithin is used in every cell of your body and is a necessary nutrient.

You can also add bran and whole seeds into the blender, and it will break them up, if it is a high speed blender.

Smoothie Recipes

So, here are a few smoothie recipes you can blend. Just use the ideas presented in the previous chapter to build up your smoothies. Drink these smoothies for breakfast or take them to work for snack time.

- Apple Smoothie

- Apple-Barley Smoothie

- Apricot Smoothie

- Peach-Rice Dream Smoothie

- Pineapple Smoothie

- Strawberry Smoothie

- Sweet-Yams-Banana Smoothie

- Papaya Smoothie

- Prune and Apple Juice Blend

- Banana Fig Smoothie

- High Fiber Breakfast Smoothie

- Mango Cool Smoothie

- Mango Passion Smoothie

- Papaya Smoothie

Apple Smoothie

Mix in the blender the following.
- 1-2 small apples cut into wedges

- 1 banana

- 1 cup 50:50 rice dream: almond milk

- ¼ cup or less of raisins soaked overnight

- 1-teaspoon honey

- 1-2 cubes of ice

- 1-teaspoon lecithin granules

- 2 teaspoons flax seed oil

Start by mixing the banana and the liquids. Then add slices of apples to get the consistency you like.

Apricot Smoothie

- One cup of fresh apricots or dried apricots that were soaked overnight

- Juice of 1/2 a lemon

- Two oz. of prune juice

- One teaspoon or more of oat ban

- One teaspoon of mineral whey

Add a slight amount of distilled water to make the consistency to your liking.

Peach-Rice Dream Smoothie

Mix in the blender:
- 2 fresh peaches with peel

- 1-cup rice dream or almond milk

- 1/2 banana

- 1-teaspoon sesame seeds

- 1-teaspoon sunflower seed

- 1-teaspoon lecithin granules

- 2 teaspoons flax seed oil

Pineapple Smoothie

Mix the following in a blender.
- 1-2 cups of fresh pineapples

- 1/2 cups apple slices

- 1/4 cup fresh apple juice

- 1/2 cup apple juice (more or less as needed)

- 1 banana

- 1-teaspoon lecithin

- 1-teaspoon flax seeds

- 2 teaspoons bran (wheat, oat or rice)

Strawberry Smoothie

Mix in a blender the following ingredients.
- 1 banana

- 1-teaspoon of lecithin granules

- 1-teaspoon of any type of bran

- 1 cup or more 50:50 rice dream: almond milk

- Now add strawberries one by one with the blender on until you get the consistency you like.

- Now in a coffee grinder, grind the following and add them to the blended strawberry mix:

- 1-teaspoon flax seeds

- 1 or 2 teaspoon sunflower seeds

- 1-teaspoon sesame seeds

Prune and Apple Juice Blend

Rinse prunes in distilled water to remove any dirt or contamination. Soak 3/4 cup or more of prunes overnight. Just slightly cover the prunes with distilled water. In the morning, blend prunes with its water and one cup of apple juice. Add a couple of slices of apple with its peel. Squeeze 1/2 lemon and blend again.

Add more apple juice to get the consistency you like. This makes a great morning drink to get your bowels moving later in the morning.

Banana Fig Smoothie

Use 1 cup of rice dream, almond milk, and soy milk mixture. You can use just one of these liquids or all combined. Add one banana and figs to get the thickness you like.

After you have blended this mixture add the following:

- 1 teaspoon of sesame seeds

- 1 teaspoon or more of lecithin

- 1 teaspoon or more of flaxseed oil

This mixture will give you many minerals and nutrients and in addition help as a natural laxative drink.

High Fiber Breakfast Smoothie
Here's a drink you can prepare in the morning and can serve as breakfast.

In a blender add,

- One half a banana that is not overripe

- One half an apple

- A few strawberries, fresh or frozen

- ¾ cup or so of rice dream, almond milk, or organic soy milk

- one rounded teaspoon of each bran - wheat, rice, and oat.

- one tablespoon of lecithin granules

- one teaspoon of flaxseed oil

- The bran will help you bulk up your stool.

Mango Cool Smoothie

Combine the following in a blender:
- One peeled and cored mango

- 1/4 to 1/2 cup of orange juice

- 1/2 banana

- a few ice cubes to give it some consistency

- teaspoon of flaxseed oil

- teaspoon to tablespoon of oat bran

- teaspoon of sesame seeds

14: Easy Exercises To Help You Lose Weight

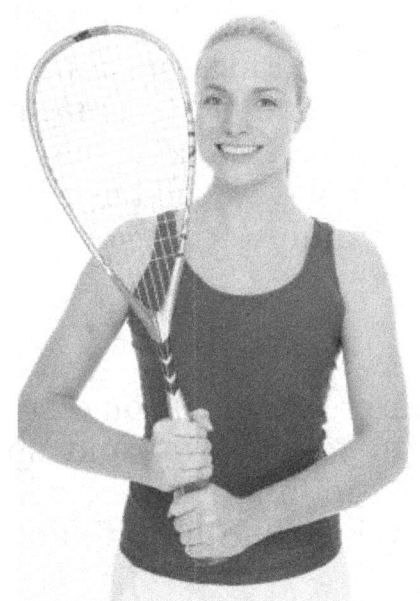

Exercise for Weight Loss

You will not lose weight if you just exercise. What is most important is what you eat. Exercising is fine tuning your weight-loss program. When you exercise and eat a good healthy diet you will lose weight.

One of the best ways to exercise to lose weight, increase your metabolism, and muscle strength is to do "interval exercise." In this process, you exercise fast in a short burst followed by a slower pace exercise or rest period and then again a fast burst.

Studies have shown that interval training will help you burn more fat and increase your metabolism than the typical lengthy steady exercises – treadmill, aerobics, bike riding, swimming, etc.

Strength training is definitely an activity that will help you reduce fat and increase muscle mall. Since muscle weighs more than fat, you may not see a quick weight loss as you gain muscle, but your body will have more energy, and you will burn more calories as you continue this training.

Walking

So what are the exercises you should be doing? There is no need to go to the gym and spend an hour running on the tread mill or riding a bike. Sure you can do these exercises, but they are not the best ones to lose weight.

If you want to walk, the walk as fast as you can for one minute, then walk slowly until your heart rate comes back to normal, then walk real fast again. Rotate from fast to slow walk for about 5 to 6 times. You can increase these frequencies as you increase your stamina.

Other Exercises

There are many other exercises that are good for you. If you play sports and like riding a bike or swimming, then this is what you should do. Doing yoga is also an excellent exercise or dancing. You pick the exercise you like to do so that you will always look forward to doing it.

The idea in losing weight is to only eat the amount of calories that your body needs or to eat just a little less than what your body needs. And, if you couple this with some exercise this will burn some more of the fat you have stored all over your body.

If you walk, walk for a comfortable distance and then either try to increase you walk every day. Or, you can walk the same distance, but walk it faster.

Rebounder

Using a rebounder is another way to exercise at home. With the rebounder you can jump up and down and help tone your muscles. In addition, you activate the lymph liquid in your body to circulate better. This is an excellent way to help your body detoxify, especially if you do this in the morning.

Actually, doing your exercise in the morning will definitely help your body detoxify and help you lose more weight.

The Pace Program

There is another program that is one of the best exercise programs that is available. It is called the "**PACE**" exercise program. You can learn more about this on the Internet. This program is great for losing weight and for strengthening your cardiovascular system.

15: Step By Step Details For Losing Weight

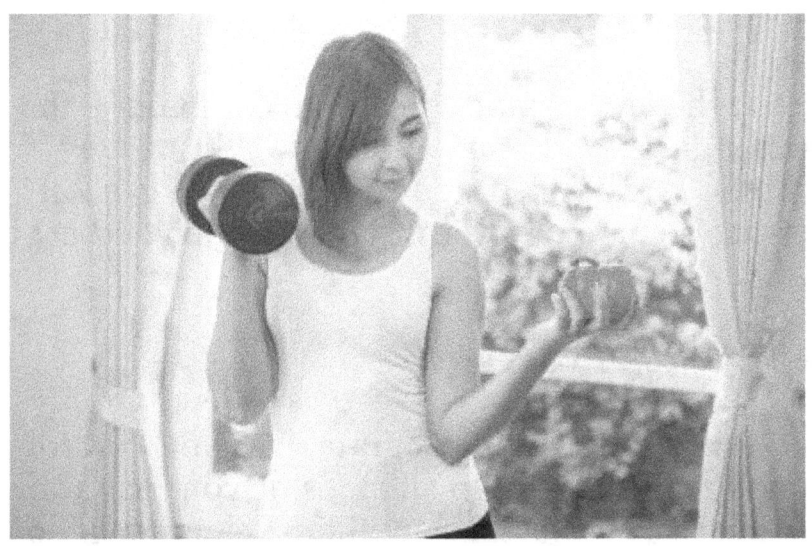

Final Comments

There you have it a method of changing your eating habits. So why change your eating habits? Because the way you have been eating has made you gain weight. This eating habits program is not a diet that you come off after you have lost weight. This program is an eating habit that you continue to use, but in a relaxed manner, so you can maintain your weight and health.

Eating differently will provide you with a different outcome – losing weight and better health.

You don't have to stop eating a lot of the things you

like you just have to eat less of them. And, you need to eat healthier food. Eating an excess of processed food is a sure way of gaining and keeping weight. This type of food has no fiber and no digestive enzymes.

Follow the cycles and the food combining that is outlined here, and you will lose weight. There are a lot of foods that are listed here that you can eat, but there are some foods that you have watch and eat less of.

Step by Step Program

Here is a step by step program that you can follow. You may not have to do all steps or you may want to do parts of it. You can buy the products you do not have, or you can use other similar products.

The main idea is to eat fewer calories, detoxify your body, eat more fruits and vegetables, alkalize your body, improve your metabolism, eat more fiber, take certain supplements, and do daily exercises.

1. Eating fewer Calories

One of the main principles in losing weight is to eat less food than your body needs. In this way, your body will start to use your fat as energy. Remember if you eat 3400 fewer calories per day, you will lose 1 pound of fat per day. But, in this program, you don't have to count calories, just start following the steps below, and you will start losing weight.

2. Body Cleanse

In any health program you start, you need to do a colon-body cleanse. It's no different here. Doing a 3, 4 or 5 day cleanse is not that difficult. You may feel reluctant to do this, but, if you want to lose weight, do the cleanse.

Chapter 5 gives you a choice of using Oxypowder or Prune juice for the cleanse. Using the Oxypowder gives you a better cleanse, but you can still get a good cleanse with prune juice.

Buy the following juices for this cleanse a few days before or the day before your cleanse.

- Organic apple juice – one gallon
- Organic apples – 3 for one day, 10 apples for three days
- Organic prune juice – 1/2 gallon
- Organic Cherry juice – 1/2 gallon
- Carrots for your juicer or carrot juice – one quart
- 4-6 Lemons

Buy other fruits you like to eat in the morning or as snacks later in the day. But try to use mostly fruit and vegetable juices without sugar.

If you have constipation, this cleanse will clear your colon of any matter you have there. Once your cleanse is over, you'll have a fresh start with your bowel movements. By eating, as outline here, you will not have trouble with constipation.

3. Body Cycles

Do the body cycles. The body cycles are an old concept that is not talked about much. But, many nutritionists are using it without really knowing where this concept originated.

Chapter 6 has a good explanation on what to do during cycles 1, 2, and 3. The most important part is cycle 1 where you only eat fruits, vegetables, and their juices in the morning. This will accelerate your weight-loss efforts.

Make the best effort to drink the recommend when you first wake up. Just choose one of these drinks before your shower or eating your fruit bowel.

4. Alkaline body

Here is another important step. Look at the best foods that make your body alkaline and incorporate them into cycle 1.

One of the best alkaline fruits is watermelon. So, make sure you eat watermelon for breakfast and breaks, when it is in season.

Likewise, use the other alkaline fruits and mix them in with other fruits or vegetables that are not so alkaline.

Eat more lemons, mangos, papaya, melons, cantaloupes, pineapples, kiwis, and raisins and dates. Use them to make smoothies.

5. Fiber

Eating 30 to 35 grams of fiber each day will make your weight-loss efforts a success. Eating 1 gm. of fiber will eliminate 8 calories from the food you eat. So eating 30 gram per day will prevent you from absorbing 240 calories from your food daily.
As you start to increase your fiber, make sure you increase your water intake to reduce any gas you may produce.

Seaweed

If you like seaweed, it has plenty of fiber. Seaweed has the fiber agar, alginates, and carrageenan. It can help you increase the feeling of satiety, just like fruits and vegetables do.

Eight grams of seaweed can give you the same amount of fiber as one banana.

In some health food stores you can find seaweed in bins, such as hijiki, wakame, kombu, nori, and kanten. Start experimenting with these, if you have not tried them.

Fruits

Take a look at the fruit fiber chart and add those fruits with the highest fiber to your cycle one breakfast. Do this for the first two weeks, then start eating some of the other fruits that have less fiber.

Start with apples, blackberries, blueberries, cantaloupes, figs, kiwis, oranges, pears, raspberries, tangerines, and watermelon.

Don't forget about the fiber in vegetables. You need to use them raw as often as you can during cycle 2 with your regular meals. Some vegetables you need to cook, but minimize the cooking time to prevent the destruction of their fiber.

6. Metabolic accelerators

There are many metabolic accelerators to use. So, just start with two a week and add more as the weeks go by.
You can start with,

- Adding chili and other spicy herbs or condiments to your food.

- Drink Green tea in the morning

- Eat 4 to 5 small meals

- Do the pace exercise three times a week.

7. Supplements

You need to take some supplements, because doing a program like this, you may not get all the nutrition you need. So start by taking the following supplements and add one of the others once a week.

B vitamin, Banaba, Digestive enzymes

Take B vitamins only with meals. Digestive enzymes can be taken before, during, or after meals. Follow the instructions on the bottle for using Banaba.

8. Smoothies

Look over the smoothie list and use one of these or one that you create. In cycle 1 breakfast, you can eat a bowl of fruit or you can use the fruit for a smoothie.

You can drink a smoothie each morning. And the left overs put in a thermos for snack breaks during the day.

Add to your smoothie other nutrients to power up your smoothie. Use ground up flax seed, sunflower seed, lecithin, a bit of honey, and powered vitamin C.

9. Exercise

Exercise is also one of the keys to losing weight. So, develop a weekly routine that you will keep. Your exercise does not have to be hours at the gym or at home watching exercise videos. The pace program gives you a 15 to 20 minute exercise routine that is more effective than other longer routines.

It does not hurt to do other physical activities that you enjoy. If you take walks or go swimming, this gives you an additional edge in your weight-loss program. You convert these activities into a pace exercise program.

If you do resistant exercise to build up your muscles, it may appear that you are not losing weight, since muscles weight more than fat.

16: About The Author And Other Resources

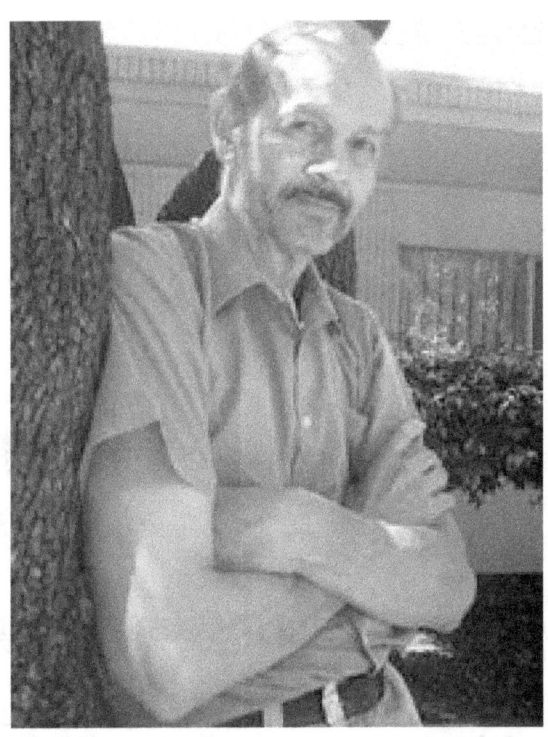

Rudy Silva is a natural consultant nutritionist educated in the United State in Nutrition and Physics. He is a graduate from San Jose State University in California. He spent 3 years undergoing psychological therapy at The Institute for Primal Therapy and an additional 5 years with a private Primal Therapy Therapist. He is author of 45 other e-books on natural remedies. He has authored a newsletter in natural remedies for over 4 years.

Resource page

Here are some of the other kindle e-books about natural remedies that have been written by this author. You can see the entire list at:

http://tinyurl.com/b2f7wd3

Acne Remedies
Best natural acne treatments: Acne facial

Constipation Remedies
Best Constipated Women Natural Cures
How To Relieve Constipation With Fruits

Essential Fatty Acids
Taking The Mystery Out Of Essential Fatty acids

Nutrition Remedies
Secret Healthy Fruit Practices Revealed
Fast Healing Juice Nutrition Therapy: Nutrition Tips 3
Calcium (Discover How To Use Calcium To Avoid Devastating Diseases)
Magnesium Nutrition Revealed
Best Nutrition Health Practices
Potassium Health Secrets Revealed
A Sodium Diet (What You Must Know About Sodium)

Stomach Remedies
Acid Reflux: Fast and Easy Cures For Acid Reflux

Asthma Treatment Cures With Remedies
How To Do Natural Colon Cleansing

Misc Remedies
Natural Hair Loss Treatment: Women And Men
Effective Natural Hemorrhoids Treatment
Iron Deficiency Anemia
Best Impotence Health Diet
What Is A Hiatus Hernia
Best Varicose Vein Treatments?

Men's Health
Best Impotence Health Diet

Weight loss
Ten (10) Day Quick Success Weight Loss Program: A new approach to losing weight by changing your eating habits for life

To see all of the kindle books written by this author, go to this the Authors Profile Page or this URL,

http://tinyurl.com/b2f7wd3

If you need support or want to promote any of his e-books, please contact him at rss41@yahoo.com and expect a reply within 24 hours. He looks forward to hearing from you and is happy to help you understand his material on natural and nutritional health.

Give A Review

And, don't for get to give a review for this e-book at Amazon, so that others can gain the benefits of what is in this e-book. A review can be a few sentences.

Rudy S. Silva, Natural Nutritionist

www.ingramcontent.com/pod-product-compliance
Lightning Source LLC
Chambersburg PA
CBHW070708290526
45790CB00001B/494